HEALTHY KNEES STRENGTH

The 4-Point Method You Need to Reduce Pain, Stabilize Your Knees, and Move with Confidence

HEALTHY KNEES STRENGTH

The 4-Point Method You Need to Reduce Pain, Stabilize Your Knees, and Move with Confidence

ROBIN ROBERTSON
WITH CO-AUTHOR TYLER BUDWEY

Niche Pressworks
INDIANAPOLIS, IN

HEALTHY KNEES STRENGTH

978-1-946533-95-1 Paperback
978-1-946533-96-8 eBook

Published by Niche Pressworks; http://NichePressworks.com

DEDICATION

Healthy Knees Strength is dedicated to all the doctors, physical therapists, fitness professionals, and other health specialists who have guided my journey through a lifetime of knee challenges and twelve knee surgeries. You have taught me so much.

I also dedicate this book to our 2019 team at the Bellingham Training and Tennis Club, for without your care and expertise in running the Club, I never could have afforded the time to write.

—Robin Robertson

To all those that have helped guide my education and decision making, as well as those that have challenged my beliefs and forced me to grow as a person.

—Tyler Budwey

TABLE OF CONTENTS

Preface   Is This Book for You?......................................ix

Chapter 1   Stopping the Spiral of Pain...........................1

Chapter 2   How My Long Hard Road
             Becomes Your Shortcut 15

Chapter 3   The Keys to Staying Fit
             and Healthy, Even with Knee Pain 23

Chapter 4   It's More Than Just Your Knee..................31

Chapter 5   Healthy Knees Strength Solution:
             Your Plan & The Exercises........................43

Chapter 6   You Have More Control Than You Think............113

Chapter 7   Moving Forward 121

About the Authors...127

IS THIS BOOK FOR YOU?

Hello! My name is Robin Robertson, and I'm excited to help you—and your knees—start feeling better. I have more personal experience with knee pain than I really want—you'll read my story in Chapter 2. That experience, along with tons of research, testing, personal results, and results from our Healthy Knees clients uniquely qualifies me to help you out.

Since 2000, I've owned and managed our family business, the Bellingham Training & Tennis Club (BTTC). My certifications in Personal Training and as a United States of America Cycling (USAC) coach give me the scientific base to work from. Plus, over 50,000 miles on a bicycle, along with 30 years of strength training with poor knees, have provided me with the practical experience that serves as the springboard to bring you great benefit.

I've been able to use BTTC as our "test kitchen" to develop programming that delivers results to our clients to reduce knee pain, get stronger, and gain confidence in their everyday movement so they can return to healthy, active lives. Our "Healthy Knees" programs have been so successful that we have written this book for you, bringing the best of strength training for knee health.

ROBIN & TYLER TOGETHER

In this book, I've teamed with Tyler Budwey, one of the smartest personal trainers I know, to refine the strength training protocol. Side note—when you see "I" in the book, that's me (Robin) talking. When you see "we," that's a blend of Tyler's and my ideas. I bring over 50 years of dealing with knee pain, my real-life experience with what works and what doesn't, along with years of research and practical experience with clients. Tyler brings his knowledge of biomechanics and the latest in science to create a bridge for those leaving physical therapy to pain-free functional movement. Together, we bring you a clear path to develop strength and reduce your knee pain.

We wrote this book to give you HOPE: Hope that life does not have to be defined by your knee pain and that there is something you can do about it to start feeling better right away.

You are not alone in your knee pain!
Knee pain is the #1 joint complaint to doctors. And no wonder! According to the American Academy of Family Physicians, knee pain affects about 25% of adults. Its prevalence has increased by almost 65% over the past 20 years, adding up to roughly four million doctor visits per year.[1] Not only are many people living with knee pain, but there are also more of us than ever before.

---

1 American Academy of Family Physicians, 2019. "Knee Pain in Adults and Adolescents: The Initial Evaluation." Accessed December 4, 2019. https://www.aafp.org/afp/2018/1101/p576.html

THIS BOOK IS FOR YOU IF...

- You can't keep up with your friends because your knees hold you back
- You are afraid that exercising could make your knee pain worse
- You've tried a few things, but nothing seems to really help
- You want your knees to feel better, but don't know where to start or what to do
- You are ready to do something and want the guidance to do the right things

That's IT! Let's work together to reduce your knee pain.

You'll need to be consistent with your effort as we guide you along the path with doing the right things at the right time to build on your successes.

I've written one other book, *Healthy Knees Cycling*, and have started the next, *Healthy Knees Total Knee Replacement*, which also may be helpful to you depending on where you are in your knee journey.

Taking care of your knees, like the rest of your health, is so worthwhile! We'll help you all along the way. In the end, you'll feel stronger and more confident in your knees so you can do the things you love.

CHAPTER 1

STOPPING THE SPIRAL OF PAIN

I bet you are familiar with the spiral of pain:

- Your knee hurts, and so you do less
- As you do less, you gain weight
- As you gain weight, moving hurts more
- And since it hurts more, you move even less
- And you gain more weight
- And your knees hurt more
- And you do even less

You are locked in this spiral of pain and fear of moving and making it worse is holding you back.

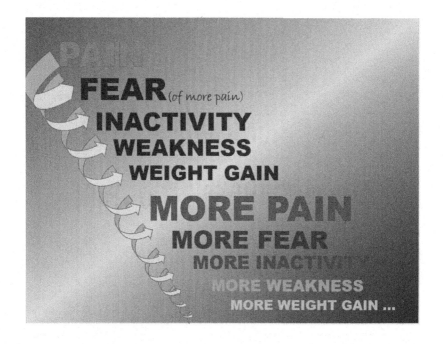

Let's dive into the pain spiral and see what's really happening here.

PAIN SPIRAL STAGE 1: PAIN REDUCES ACTIVITIES

The first part of the pain spiral is where you start moving differently and then start giving up the things you love.

Changing how you move

Your body is smart! Your brain, muscles, and bones all work together so you can move. Your body is a very good communicator, and sometimes you don't even realize you've made adjustments to how you stand, run, walk, or climb stairs.

You can still do the things you need to, even if your muscles and joints are not functioning the way they should. You might find that, because of your knee pain, you take stairs one at a time. Or maybe you walk with a limp. Or you've shortened your stride while walking. Or maybe your posture is changing; you no longer stand up straight and are starting to lean to one side or hinge forward at your hips.

The human body is constantly being shaped and re-modeled through the biomechanical forces (how your muscles and bones interact with movement and gravity) and biofeedback (does it hurt, or does it feel good?).

Your body automatically starts protecting your site of pain, so you start moving differently. This reaction to pain may reshape your body for the worse.

Compensating with other muscles or joint movements
Compensation is your body's attempt to make up for lack of movement (or avoidance of pain) in one area by recruiting movement in another area. Your brain figures out another path to achieve the movement through an altered neuromuscular strategy that fires muscles and/or structures (bones, tendons, ligaments, joints) in a different pattern.

Does this sound familiar? It used to be just your knee that gave you pain, but now your opposite hip hurts—or your low back or your ankle or even up into your shoulders.

If a doctor, therapist, or personal trainer were to watch your movement, they might detect the movement pattern changes you've made. It's their role to prescribe exercises that will strengthen your weak areas. Knee pain in the first place can be caused by many things, including compensation movements caused by weak muscles. Strength is definitely what we will help you with in this book!

Here are a couple of things to look out for with compensating movement:[2]

Chronic muscle tightness

If a muscle is working overtime, it may feel tight. Stretching may not be the entire solution. The key is to find what is WEAK that is causing the muscle to work harder. The solution lies in strengthening the weak muscle or joint.

Unusual tenderness in some muscles

Maybe you have one specific spot that is always sore. This sore spot may be caused by overworking a muscle, some change in your regular movement patterns, or even tenderness from post-exercise muscle soreness after a harder-than-usual workout. If this specific tenderness continues, it is a good idea to become more aware of how you move to see if you notice any compensation or weaknesses. Of course, it helps to work with a personal trainer or physical therapist to identify specifics.

One muscle that always seems sore

Again, this is likely a problem caused by overuse or a weak muscle. If you are overusing, it means you are depending more on this muscle to take up the slack from your weak point. Or it may be that the sore muscle is the weak muscle. For example, the feeling of

---

2 Fleet Feet, 2019, "Compensation Patterns: Your Body is Telling You Something!" Accessed December 5, 2019. https://www.fleetfeet.com/s/hartford/sports%20medicine/%20 compensation%20patterns

"tight" hamstrings can often be the result of weak hamstrings. This perception of tightness is from neurological guarding—your body trying to protect itself. This can also happen with tendinopathy, where weak muscles result in chronic overload of the tendon. The key in all these cases is to find the weak area and strengthen it.

Same recurring injury
If you have a recurring injury, there is some underlying cause that has not been addressed.

Compounding pains
Ever notice that you have a pain in one place, and then a second location pops up? Maybe it's a pain that starts in your knee, then is added to by a pain in your low back, or your opposite hip, or your calf.

Your body is working hard to find its new workaround to avoid pain. But by doing this, it may put stress in new places that can cause additional pain or discomfort. Again, the best solution is to find the underlying weakness that may be the root of these compensations.

Giving up things you love
Impact activities are usually the first to go. When talking about knees and impact, we are referring to the force that goes through the joint caused by your foot striking the ground.

In a strong, healthy knee, these impact forces are easily absorbed without pain. When you have a weakness or injury, you might think otherwise.

There are also shear forces through the knee caused by gravity and resistance (like slowing down or coming to a sudden stop). You may feel these shear forces as pain when walking up or down a hill, up or down stairs.

Impact plus shear forces put a lot of stress on the knee. In a healthy, strong knee, this is okay, no problem. But for many of us, sports that involve running with a quick change in direction, such as tennis, soccer, or basketball, may cause pain.

Maybe even before you consciously realize it, you start making changes.

Maybe you reduce the number of times per week that you go for a run.

Or when going on a walk with a friend, you choose a flat route. Next you choose a flat route with level footing, like sidewalks instead of trails, because that uneven footstep can tweak your knee.

Or you may even consciously stop doing a sport because it becomes more painful than fun. That's what happened with me and downhill skiing.

Or even, perhaps, you have a doctor tell you that if you want to preserve your knees, you need to make some immediate changes to your activities.

Little by little, you start letting go of some of the activities you've loved. Until...what's left?

PAIN SPIRAL STAGE 2: FEAR OF MOVEMENT

You've already stopped doing some of the things you love because of pain. Now you simply become afraid to move at all.

You've done this before, and then it happens. TWEAK! You get white-hot, shooting pain. Or maybe you've simply been out enjoying life, and the next day your knees are killing you. You start to become afraid of doing something that will make your knees mad, and so you start doing less and less.

Not knowing what is safe
Part of the fear of movement is not knowing what movement is safe. Some of that may stem from old habits with movements done the wrong way.

The good news is the problem might be in your form, not the movement. Before you throw the sport out the window, let's get into the basics and re-learn, re-train for proper biomechanical movement and then see how it feels.

Not knowing where to start
Being afraid of hurting more may prevent you from starting at all. Besides, you might not be quite sure where to start anyway. That's why we break down movements to get to the essential elements. Make sure those feel good and manageable before you move to the next level.

Increased inactivity can add more pain
Are your knees achy? Achy when you go to stand up after sitting a while? Does it take you a few steps to loosen up?

As your knee becomes less active, it becomes less healthy. Inside your knee joint capsule, you have a substance called "synovial fluid." The job of the synovial fluid is to nourish your cartilage and buffer some of the impact forces in the joint, as well as to lubricate movement. It's like the oil for your hinge. When the hinge (your knee) is not used regularly, or you have some osteoarthritis going on (or both), your synovial fluid may get thinner and less effective at doing its job.

I call this the "rusty hinge syndrome," and if you've had it, you know that sounds exactly how it feels.

Can you do anything about this? Yes, indeed! Regular movement, especially movement that is no impact and not weight-bearing, can be a huge benefit to your knees.

In addition to this book, I strongly urge you to follow the advice in the Healthy Knees Cycling book for the full picture of taking care of your knees. You can find more information at www.HealthyKneesBook.com.

PAIN SPIRAL STAGE 3: LOSING MUSCLE AND SLOWING METABOLISM

Simply said: use it or lose it!

Without using your muscles, your body adapts

Your body is really smart and works hard to conserve energy. So, if you have more muscle mass than you are using, your body eventually breaks it down. That means less energy is spent on supporting unused muscles. Muscle atrophy can occur for many reasons, one of them being long periods of inactivity.

The good news is that this kind of muscle atrophy can be reversed by increased activity and intentional strength-building movements. You can build muscle at just about any age!

Many research studies show the benefits of weight training at any age. My favorite is the study led by Mikel Izquierdo-Redín, Professor of Physiotherapy at the NUP/UPNA-Public University of Navarre, published in *Age*, the journal of the American Ageing Association. This study focused on weight training for a group of people over 90 years old! Yes! OVER 90 years old!

In 2013, 24 people between the ages of 91 and 96 participated in the study for 12 weeks, with 11 people in the experimental group and 13 in the control group. The experimental group trained twice per week, with various strength and balance exercises. The results showed that the experimental group improved their strength, power, and muscle mass.

So, no excuses! If an "over 90-year-old" can do this, so can you! And we will show you how.

Reducing weight-bearing movement can increase the risk of bone loss (osteoporosis)
Newton was right! Let's consider his 3rd law: for every action, there is an equal and opposite reaction. But what does this have to do with your bones and osteoporosis?

Let's first tackle osteoporosis: osteoporosis literally means porous bone (think Swiss cheese). Our bodies are constantly trying to maintain a balance. As one thing is needed here, it is taken from there, which can be the cause of osteoporosis. Two essential minerals for bone formation are calcium and phosphate. Calcium is also needed for proper functioning of the brain, heart, and other organs. If there is not enough calcium from your diet, your body may reabsorb calcium from your bones and redistribute it to maintain blood calcium levels to keep these critical organs functioning properly.[3] But this may mean that your bones become weaker!

Ask your doctor about a test for your calcium levels as supplements are available. In addition to maintaining a healthy level of calcium, putting demands on your bones through weight-bearing activity will strengthen them. This is where Newton's 3rd law comes in. As your muscles tug on your bones, your bones tug back! This makes your bones stronger.

Muscles act like pulleys to pull your bones one way or the other, creating movement. Muscles are attached to bones by tendons. As the muscle and tendon pull on the bone, the bone reacts and sends a signal to the brain that the bone needs to be strong to withstand the pull.

Weight-bearing and resistance exercises are the best for strengthening bones. Weight-bearing forces you to work against gravity with activities like walking, hiking, jogging, and dancing. Resistance exercises, such as lifting weights, can also strengthen bones.

Loss of muscle can cause you trouble in many ways:

---

3 National Osteoporosis Foundation, 2020. "What is Osteoporosis and What Causes It?" Accessed January 4, 2020. https://www.nof.org/patients/what-is-osteoporosis/

Loss of muscle slows your metabolism
Metabolism is the process through which your body turns the food you eat into the energy you need. This brings us back around to "use it or lose it." You've probably heard that your metabolism slows down with age. This is due primarily to two factors: changes in resting metabolic rate (RMR) and activity energy expenditures.[4]

Your resting metabolic rate is the rate your body burns calories when at complete rest. It's your minimum caloric need to support basic life functions. That is dependent, in part, on how much lean muscle mass you have, among many other factors. The more muscle you have, the higher your RMR and caloric needs.

When you reduce activity, you not only reduce your energy needs, but also your body reabsorbs muscle tissue that is not needed. That means you get a little weaker, and as your requirements for fuel are reduced, your metabolism slows.

So, what if your metabolism slows? If your metabolism is slowing and you don't adjust your diet, you'll likely put on weight. And weight gain can lead to more knee pain.

Loss of muscle equals less support for your joint.
If you lose muscle, it just makes everything more challenging! You have less strength for things like walking up and down stairs or even just getting out of a chair. Staying strong has everything to do with maintaining independence of movement.

---

4 PMC US National Library of Medicine, National Institutes of Health, 2010. "Energy Expenditure and Aging." https://www.ncbi.nlm.nih.gov/pmc/articles/PMC2818133/

Remember that your muscles are like pulleys to your bones. If you have a little tiny pulley, you will not be able to move that joint very well. And you may feel more pain in your joint. This can be caused by a stronger muscle overcompensating for a weak one' causing a malalignment somewhere in the knee bending and straightening process.

Loss of muscle can lead to trouble with balance

Have you ever noticed that your balance isn't as good as it used to be? I sure noticed that myself!

Practicing balance is one of the very important things you can do to improve your knee health. If all your muscles are firing and working together to keep you upright, your likelihood of falling is reduced. We'll talk about ways to practice your balance later in this book.

More muscle mass does not necessarily mean your balance will be improved, but it will provide the opportunity to have more control.

Unknown muscle loss and slower metabolism can lead to weight gain.

It might be that you are staying relatively the same "size"—but as you've lost muscle, you are adding fat, because you haven't changed your eating habits. Or maybe you notice that your clothes are not fitting the same anymore because one pound of fat takes up more space than one pound of muscle.

The problem is that as you become more sedentary, your body needs fewer calories. But you don't realize this and go on eating the same amount of food, maybe even more, because you feel so terrible about yourself and you start eating your feelings (that's a whole other book right there.) And as you gain more weight, everything hurts more.

PAIN SPIRAL STAGE 4: WEIGHT GAIN LEADS TO MORE PAIN

Why does gaining weight make your knees hurt more? That is easy to explain. For every extra pound you carry, you increase the magnitude of the loads across the knee. As you walk, run, or jump, the forces transmitted are multiplied by your body weight:

- Walking 2-3 x bodyweight[5]
- Jogging 4-5 x bodyweight
- Running 6-14 x bodyweight[6]
- Jumping 9-10+ x bodyweight

Just think, if you are carrying an extra 10 pounds, that means 20-30 MORE pounds of force through your knee when you are walking. If you have an extra 50 pounds, that's an added 100-150 pounds of force. You get the idea: more bodyweight equals more force, and that can add up to a lot more stress on your joint and more pain.

---

5 PMC US National Library of Medicine, National Institutes of Health, 2013. "Knee Joint Forces: Prediction, Measurement, and Significance." Accessed December 6, 2019. https://www.ncbi.nlm.nih.gov/pmc/articles/PMC3324308/

6 Medscape.com, 2015. "Joint Loading in Runners Does Not Initiate Knee Osteoarthritis." Accessed December 6, 2019. http://www.azisks.com/wp-content/uploads/2017/04/Joint-Loading-in-Runners-Does-Not-Initiate-Knee-Osteoarthritis.pdf

Pain spiral stages worsen as they repeat: more pain leads to less activity

More pain with movement inspires exactly no one to move more. Then you get stuck. You are in a spiral of knee pain: reducing activity, losing muscle, gaining weight, and hurting even more. That pain spiral just keeps on getting worse with every pound you gain. Your knees get achier because they're not being used, and you are locked in fear that what you try might make them worse.

Let's STOP the pain spiral!

It's time to put a stop to this pain spiral right now! With the right kind of movement and the right kind of strength training, we can pull you out of this spiral back into the land where movement feels good again. Sound good? OK, let's keep going.

CHAPTER 2

HOW MY LONG HARD ROAD BECOMES YOUR SHORTCUT

I know all about knee pain, and that's why I wanted to help you with this book. My knees have always hurt. Spoiler alert: I've had a total of 12 knee surgeries (eight on my left and four on my right), and now both knees have been replaced. I'm hoping that with the replacements, I won't see the scalpel end of a surgeon for many, many years to come. But why 12 knee surgeries?

You see, I was born with a rare congenital condition in my knees called "discoid meniscus." That was finally diagnosed after many doctor visits and cortisone shots before I was a teenager. The condition meant I had a thicker disc-shaped meniscus cartilage (instead of the normal crescent shape) in the outsides of my knees (lateral compartments). You'd think that would be a good thing, right? More cartilage equals more cushion, right? People with discoid meniscus may never have any problems with it[7]...but that wasn't my case.

---

7 American Academy of Orthopaedic Surgeons, 2019. "Diseases and Conditions: Discoid Meniscus." Accessed January 4, 2020. https://orthoinfo.aaos.org/en/diseases--conditions/discoid-meniscus

Nope. I had my first open knee surgery at age 13 to remove all of the lateral meniscus in my left knee—because that was the technology at the time. Then my doctor told me to exercise as tolerated by pain. What is that supposed to mean? For a girl who knew knee pain all of her life, it meant there would be more knee pain, but my knee would no longer lock up or give out.

So, what is a teenager to do? I became a competitive runner in high school and college, not understanding the damage I was doing by running on a knee with no meniscus cartilage. Yes, it hurt, but that was the norm. I look back at pictures of my running days and often see my knee wrapped.

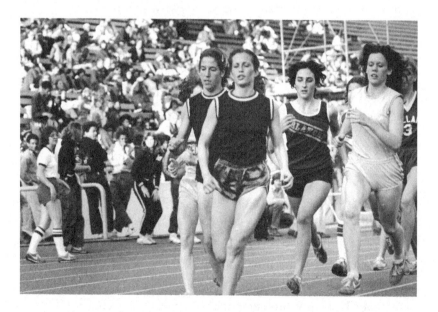

As I went into college, I was still running and downhill skiing and loving every minute of the thrill, even though there was so much pain.

The first to go for me was downhill skiing. I LOVED skiing the moguls (a series of snow bumps to ski around on a steep slope), with that feeling of thrill at the top of the run as you pick a good line, the sprinkle of snow that lifts to your face as you carve each corner, and the feeling of flow as your body moves in sync over and around each mogul with the breathless satisfaction at the bottom of the hill as you gaze up at the snowfield you just conquered.

It was a beautiful thing until the third or fourth run when my knees would scream at me, swell up, and I'd be hobbled for a week. I was 23 years old when I chose to give up skiing because it was too painful.

I had been a competitive runner since my sophomore year in high school. In the fall, I ran cross-country. I loved running those trails through the woods in the crisp days of autumn, with the crunch of leaves underfoot and the earthy smell of forest as I used mental toughness and physical training to do my best.

In the spring came track. I was a mid-distance gal, focusing on the 800M and 1500M. I loved the intensity of shoulder to shoulder competition, the strategy of the race, and the sheer willpower to dig deep and finish strong.

At 24 years old, during the winter of my senior year in college, my left knee was bad enough that I had my second surgery. I got the devastating news that I had severe osteoarthritis, and my doctor told me that if I wanted to walk when I was 30, I needed to stop all impact sports immediately.

What a blow! I was crushed. I had to drop off the track team and quit running. Despite wanting to wallow in sorrow at this loss, I knew I couldn't just throw in the towel. Ever the optimist, I had to find something else I could do that wouldn't further damage my knees and cause so much pain. I traded in my running shoes and skis and started riding my bike. It was a great solution since it was no impact, not weight-bearing and had no lateral movement. Cycling definitely saved me physically and mentally.

But that didn't mean the end of giving up activities due to knee pain, either. Hiking was the next to go. For a long time, I could hike on flats and even uphill, but like with skiing, the downhill was a killer. Just the uneven nature of the path became a showstopper. Does that sound familiar? So, I stopped hiking.

Then I began to sacrifice anything lateral movement. Side to side shuffle? Nope. Karaoke steps that you do in aerobics classes, like side-stepping with one leg crossing in front of the other? No way. It all aggravated my knees.

Even swimming became a problem for me because my left knee had become "loose." This happened because I was becoming very "knock-kneed" as my lateral compartment compressed. That meant there was some looseness in the joint since one of the collateral ligaments was stretching out, and the other was slack. I'd kick, and my knee would wobble and felt like it wasn't connecting right. Ouch!

And then came stairs—the pain with descending, ultimately followed by pain going upstairs as well. To avoid it, you start "2 stepping"—one leg does the work, and the other follows. Have you ever had that happen?

Just walking was no longer comfortable.

Even standing still for more than 15 minutes was aggravating and painful.

But here was the bigger problem. It wasn't even just about me. My knee pain also defined my children's lives.

At 34 years old, I could hardly walk around the block or stand for any length of time, but worse yet, I could not keep up with my kids.

This really hit home when my kids were just two and four years old. I could no longer take them to the park because I couldn't keep up with them when they ran around. I couldn't chase after them. I could not keep them safe.

That broke my heart and forced my hand to my next surgery. I already needed a knee replacement, but no doctor would consent to perform that procedure on a 34-year-old because, at that time, a knee replacement was estimated to last 20 years, and they thought it could be replaced two times. That only got me to my early 70's— then what? There was no continuing solution. This prospect scared me deeply and helped me to understand that taking care of my knees was imperative. It was then that I decided to do everything I could to fight for and protect my knees.

Instead of replacement, I had a leg reconstruction surgery (oste-otomy) that re-aligned my leg so that I was no longer knock-kneed. This was intended to reduce my pain, slow the degeneration, and buy me more time before the ultimate replacement.

Since that time, there were many more knee surgeries to trim out remaining bits of frayed cartilage, to remove floating "kibbles and bits," and to even shave down bone spurs related to my advancing arthritis.

Because of my commitment to doing the very best for my knees (all the right things I describe in this book for you), I was able to delay the first replacement for 26 years, far longer than the seven to ten years predicted from the osteotomy. It was quite traumatic for me to finally decide to replace. I'd have to say goodbye to my own bones that I fought so hard to protect. I actually mourned the loss of my natural knees and worried that replacements would not turn out better than what I was leaving behind. I was scared.

Ultimately, the arthritis, damage to my bones, degrading leg alignment, compensating movements, and constant pain led me to replace both of my knees (two years apart). The results from my first total knee replacement (TKR) were so positive that I had far fewer concerns about replacing my other knee. I'm now back to full speed with strength training, biking, and I am looking forward to hikes that I could never have done pre-TKR. I feel strong, able, and ready, and I want to help you feel that way too.

So how does one stay healthy and fit with all these challenges?

It is a choice.

A choice to find a way around the roadblock. You've got to decide that the outcome you want is worth the effort of transition. You've got to want it more than you are afraid of it. You have to believe that what you do will make a difference. And you have to do the work.

This book distills all I have learned over the many years of knee pain, surgeries, and recoveries to give you the shortcut to taking care of your knees now. You, too, can make that choice to improve your knees and improve your health. You can do this!

CHAPTER 3

THE KEYS TO STAYING FIT AND HEALTHY, EVEN WITH KNEE PAIN

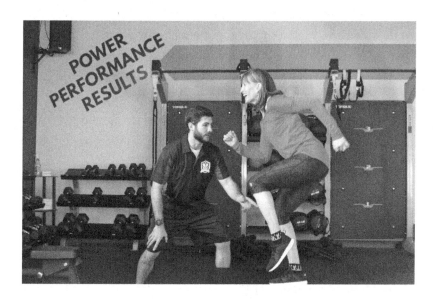

The condition of your knees may not be your fault, **but it is your problem**.

So, what do we do about this?

Our goal is to help you preserve, strengthen, and use your knees as long as possible. Elective surgery should be the last resort after you've tried all of the other things (as your condition allows) to get stronger and more stable.

After my surgeon told me that I would have had my knees replaced more than a decade ago, if it weren't for riding a bike (and strength training), I knew I was onto something. I put all that knowledge of how to make it work into our Healthy Knees programs.

We've had clients go through our Healthy Knees programs who had knee surgery planned, but after completing the work with us, they canceled their surgery and never looked back. And, sure, some still needed surgery, but they went into the surgery stronger, so they had a better starting place for recovery.

Here's the key: do the work first. Get as strong as you can. And even if you still need surgery, you will be at a much better place for recovery.

There are three main keys to staying fit and healthy even with knee pain, and each one unlocks new possibilities for you. You need all three to keep your knees at their peak condition:

1. Joint movement with low or no impact cardio activities
2. Strength to support knee and body movement
3. Consistency and can-do attitude

1. Joint movement with low or no impact cardio activities

Moving your knee the right way is important to maintain healthy function. Achy knees with little activity can start to feel like that rusty hinge. Knees that have taken a pounding from sports can feel painfully abused. We want you to get moving in a way that works the knee but doesn't irritate it. That's why we recommend low and no impact activities for your knees.

If you have been sedentary, activities like cycling, swimming, or using an elliptical are wonderful places to start (with my preference being bicycling). All three of these options provide ways to work your knee range of motion and leg muscles while offering the opportunity to work on your cardio (heart) fitness as well.

If you are a runner or avid hiker (or some other impact sport) and not yet ready to give it all up, simply swap out one or two days per week with riding a bike, swimming, or using an elliptical machine.

Why a bike?
A bicycle offers you a no-impact, no weight-bearing, no lateral movement way to move your knee joint and exercise your legs (and your heart). Motion is lotion! The movement helps your knee function better. You can do bicycling indoor on a stationary bike or outside while you see the world. Either way is a great way to exercise. Sure, your bum will have to get used to the seat, but after two to four weeks, it's not so noticeable.

It does take 110 degrees of bend in the knee to be able to pedal a bike. If you have a range less than that, biking might not be for you just now. This is also why bike set up is extremely important as a part of protecting your knees (seat position) and for comfort (handlebar position).

If you want to learn more about riding a bike the right way to help your knees, I recommend that you read my book *Healthy Knees Cycling* for all of the details.

Why swimming?

Swimming is another no weight-bearing and no-impact activity that is a full-body workout. The water supports your weight and provides resistance immediately. If you are not a swimmer, you can use the pool for "running" while wearing floats. You may feel some of the lateral movement through your knees during different kinds of swimming kicks. You'll have to judge whether or not that feels comfortable for you.

Why an elliptical machine?

An elliptical machine simulates running with very low impact and no lateral movement. The footpads of the elliptical machine support your feet as you simulate a walk or run. You are challenged to do some weight-bearing, which is good for building bone density but can be uncomfortable for your knees.

2. Strength to support knee and body movement

The cardio activities listed above address reducing stress in your knees and getting stronger in ways specific to each sport. But they do not address all of the muscles you need to have the healthiest knees overall. This is why adding our 4-point method for knee strength to your exercise program is an important step to overall knee health. The point of strength training is not really about lifting weights; it's about reducing physical stresses and preparing your body for the things you want to DO in life.

We show you through Movement Foundations how proper technique will preserve your knees.

I often hear "I can't squat" when a client first comes to our Healthy Knees programs. By the end of our time together, they surprise themselves that with the proper technique, they actually CAN squat. This essential motion isn't just for strength, as you know if you live with pain. A squat is how you do things like getting on and off a chair (or toilet) with ease, picking up a bag of groceries from the floor, lowering down to dig out those pesky weeds in your garden, and even getting on and off the floor more comfortably.

Whether you are moving in everyday life or doing specific weight-lifting activities, proper form is king. Good ankle, knee, and hip alignment may change a painful move into one that feels okay.

When your muscles are stronger, movement is easier. To make your muscles stronger, you must give them a challenge. This principle is called "overload," which may sound bad and like you are overdoing it. But what it really means is that the intensity of the exercise must be high enough above normal for physiological adaptation to occur.[8]

8 International Sports Science Association, 2020. "Understanding and Using the Overload Principle." Accessed January 4, 2020. https://www.issaonline.com/blog/index.cfm/2019/understanding-and-using-the-overload-principle

That is how you get stronger! Your body will change when your muscles are taxed to the point where they must grow stronger in order to respond to the demand of lifting weights.

Have no fear; you will not start with lifting some giant dumbbell. No, instead, we will begin at the beginning with bodyweight exercises so that you learn proper technique. And if you've never lifted weights, bodyweight exercises will be plenty. It is enough to activate movement in a way you haven't done before.

Once the bodyweight exercises seem easy, it is time to start adding to the challenge with weights. You might be surprised to find out how empowered you feel as you get stronger lifting heavier and heavier weights. It feels good to be strong!

Why does strength matter?

It comes down to one word: Independence. Being strong and able will keep you independent.

Muscle strength is important for maintaining your independence—simply being able to complete basic life activities (getting out of a chair, climbing stairs, walking around without falling).

Perhaps you are looking beyond independence to regaining some of your life's joys, such as going for walks with your friends and being able to keep up or playing with your grandkids on the floor without needing help to stand back up. Perhaps you have loftier goals like hiking a challenging route in a beautiful part of the world or riding your bike on an adventure tour.

If you are like me, the main point is that you want to be ready. Ready to say YES to things you love in life without being afraid that you can't do them.

Now, of course, there may be some things you'll wisely say no to because it's not in the best interest of your knees. For me, that means I will never run again or take up the sport of tennis. But I will be able to say YES to hikes and bike rides. In fact, my husband and I are riding our bikes across the country in 3-week sections at a time. Do you know how good it feels to say YES to that? It is amazing!

I want to empower you to say YES to trying new things and return to the things that are important to you.

3. Consistency and can-do attitude

Now that I've gotten you all fired up to say YES to the things you want to do in life, we must talk about the third key to staying fit and healthy: consistency and can-do attitude.

Many people ask me how I stay in such great shape even with all my knee surgeries. My answer is that I am consistent. You just have to keep at it. Some days you may not feel like doing anything at all, and the important thing will be just to get started. A little bit is better than nothing.

To get results, you've got to do the work regularly, to have consistency. This is a fix that can last the rest of your life as long as you keep doing the work. It's a little like brushing your teeth; you can't save it up; you have to brush regularly to get the results.

Taking care of your body is something that needs attention and respect consistently.

How often? We recommend a minimum of two times a week strength training and two times a week low impact cardio training as your base. When you start, you can even do the strength and cardio on the same day. If you truly want to make a difference with your knees, you can definitely fit this into your life.

We are so excited for you to start this journey of great knee health. Not only do we believe in you, but more importantly, we want you to believe in yourself—your attitude matters. What you say to yourself makes a difference with how things turn out.

I heard a saying once, "What you think is where you go," and find that to be so true. If you think you can, you are way more likely to succeed than if you think you can't. Believing you can make a difference in your body and your health is a very powerful part of your success.

YES! You can do this! You can create the habit and lifestyle that includes your knee exercises, and you will see results so you can do the things in life you love.

CHAPTER 4

IT'S MORE THAN JUST YOUR KNEE

Your knee health is about more than just the muscles attached directly to your knee. It's about how your knee works as part of your whole-body system.

It is time for a brief anatomy lesson so you can see how it all fits together.

Anatomy of the Right Knee[9]

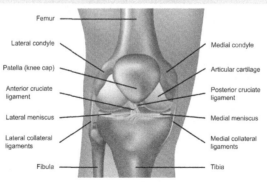

Femur
Lateral condyle
Patella (knee cap)
Anterior cruciate ligament
Lateral meniscus
Lateral collateral ligaments
Fibula
Medial condyle
Articular cartilage
Posterior cruciate ligament
Medial meniscus
Medial collateral ligaments
Tibia

9 Graphic license Dreamstime 25432096

KNEE JOINT—how it works

The knee is a modified hinge joint that allows flexion and extension. It's called "modified" because there is slight internal and external rotation as you bend and straighten your knee. When you bend your knee, the end of the femur bone rocks over the meniscus cartilage and tibia. Your knee is a synovial joint because of the joint capsule that holds in the lubricating synovial fluid that reduces the friction when you move (remember the "rusty hinge").

Bones of the knee and leg

Three bones meet to form your knee: femur (thigh bone), tibia (the shin bone), and patella (kneecap).

Your lower leg also has a smaller bone, the fibula. This smaller of the two lower leg bones is nestled to the lateral side of your tibia. It sits underneath the tibial plateau and is not considered part of the knee joint.

At the foot end of your shin, your tibia and fibula connect to the bones of your foot. Your outside ankle bone is the end of your fibula.

At the hip end of your leg, your femur is attached to your pelvic bone in the ball and socket joint of your hip.

Cartilage—the protection for your bones

Your knee has two types of cartilage: meniscus (fibrocartilage) and articular cartilage.

Meniscus Cartilage

The real cushions of the knee are the two C-shaped menisci cartilage, which sit on the tibial plateau between the femur and tibia. The menisci act as shock absorbers and are made of dense fibrocartilage that is sort of like memory foam. The cartilage continually changes shape to adapt to the movement of the knee but returns to its original shape. The menisci also help to stabilize the knee in medial and lateral movements (side to side).

Articular Cartilage

Articular cartilage is like shrink-wrap padded protection for the ends of your bones, generally 2-4 mm thick[10]. The knee side of your patella has the thickest articular cartilage in your whole body at up to 7mm thick. This thick cartilage helps to dissipate large joint reaction forces that are created during forceful contractions of the quadriceps muscle, like when you kick a ball.[11]

Ligaments—the "ropes" that tie bones together

Ligaments are made of dense connective tissue. They connect bone to bone, whereas tendons connect muscle to bone.

The most famous of your knee ligaments are the cruciate ligaments. Inside the knee joint are the two ligaments, crossing each other like an "X," connecting the femur to the tibia.

---

10 National Center for Biotechnology Information, 2009. *Journal of Sports Health*, "The Basic Science of Articular Cartilage." Accessed January 4, 2020. https://www.ncbi.nlm.nih.gov/pmc/articles/PMC3445147/

11 National Center for Biotechnology Information, 2016. *International Journal of Sports Physical Therapy*, "Biomechanics and Pathomechanics of the Patellofemoral Joint." Accessed January 4, 2020. https://www.ncbi.nlm.nih.gov/pmc/articles/PMC5095937/

The Anterior Cruciate Ligament (ACL) is toward the front of the knee, and the Posterior Cruciate Ligament (PCL) is behind it. Tears to the ACL are often seen in sports injuries. Besides keeping your bones connected and in place, your ACL is responsible for preventing your knee from "hyperextension" or your knee bending backward the wrong way. The PCL's job is to prevent "hyperflexion" (too much bend in the knee) and displacement by your thigh bone (femur) moving too far forward over your tibia or your tibia moving too far backward.

The other ligaments of your knee include the collateral ligaments on the sides. These provide stability and brace your knee against unusual movement. The lateral (fibular) collateral ligament stabilizes the outside.

The medial (tibial) collateral ligament (MCL) reinforces the inside of your knee. The MCL is also connected to your medial meniscus. An injury to this ligament usually affects the medial meniscus as well.

Damage to the collateral ligaments can be caused by a force that pushes the knee sideways and is often, but not always a direct contact injury[12] (football, hockey) or movements that require a quick change in direction (soccer, basketball).

---

12 Ortho Info and the Academy of Orthopaedic Surgeons, 2014. "Collateral Ligament Injuries." Accessed January 31, 2020. https://orthoinfo.aaos.org/en/diseases--conditions/collateral-ligament-injuries/

What's a kinetic chain, and why does it matter?
You know that song, "Dem Bones"?

The leg bone's connected to the knee bone,
The knee bone's connected to the thigh bone,
The thigh bone's connected to the hip bone...

That's essentially the kinetic chain! A little more scientifically speaking, the kinetic chain describes all of the body parts that work together to create movement. The lower kinetic chain includes the toes, feet, ankles, lower legs, upper legs, hips, pelvis, and spine.

People often assume that when their knee hurts, it's all about the knee. But it is wise to look at the whole kinetic chain to see if there is a weakness or imbalance elsewhere.

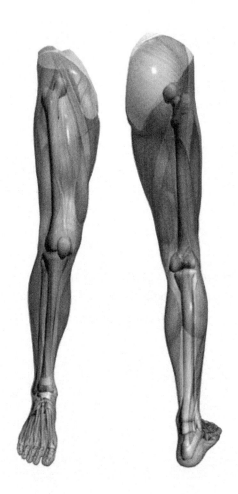

Pictured: Muscles and bones of front right leg and back of right leg[13]

We'll start at the end of the kinetic chain (feet) and work our way up to your core.

---

13 Left: Front of leg (anterior); Right back of leg (posterior). Photo licenses Dreamstime: anterior leg file ID 201234, posterior leg File ID 201235

Toes/Feet/Ankles

One common contributor to knee pain is one that people least expect: the feet![14] Your foot is crazy complicated with 28 bones, 30 joints, and more than 100 muscles, tendons, and ligaments—all linked together to provide support, balance, and mobility.[15]

If your feet roll inward or outward too far, it can cause the lower leg to move in a way that creates stress in the knee on every step.

Shoes are another important matter. Poor-fitting or worn-out footwear can cause a malalignment that contributes to knee pain. The amount of support you want or need in a shoe can depend on many things. "Barefoot" style shoes have less padding and support and generally ask your feet to do more work. If you want to wear this style, make sure you allow for a break-in period, so your feet muscles don't get overworked.

The more support and cushion your shoes provide, the less work your foot has to do with balance and movement. Shoe inserts, or orthotics, may be a good temporary addition to your footwear while you work on strengthening areas that contribute to your individual issue.

Think of your feet as your foundation. If your feet are not firmly planted on the ground, your foundation is off. Weak foot muscles, paired with tight calf muscles, can mess with your gait and foot

---

14 Pedorthic Association of Canada, 2019. "If your knees hurt take a look at your feet." Accessed December 8; 2019. https://www.pedorthic.ca/ if-your-knees-hurt-take-a-look-at-your-feet/

15 Arthritis Foundation Anatomy of the Foot. Accessed January 4, 2020. https://www.arthritis.org/about-arthritis/where-it-hurts/foot-heel-and-toe-pain/foot-anatomy.php

alignment,[16] and that may throw off leg alignment. All this adds up to pitching you forward or backward. If your base becomes tilted (feet and leg alignment), you can see from there how that will negatively affect your overall posture

If your toes, feet, or ankles are weak or limited in flexibility, it will affect not only your walking gait, but may also be the root cause of difficulty performing squatting movements, like sitting down or standing up from a chair or getting on and off the toilet.

Your proprioceptive nerves help you understand your motion and body position in space. Proprioception is sometimes called your "6th sense" and is vital for maintaining balance. Proprioceptive nerve endings are present in your muscles and tendons and help coordinate body movements.

Your feet are one of three anatomical regions, along with the spine and cervical spine, supplied with more proprioceptive nerves than other parts of your body.[17] Shoes with heavy support can limit or mask your foot's ability to sense through proprioception.

If you choose to transition from a highly supportive shoe toward one with minimal support or even the "barefoot" style of shoe, make that transition through stages so that your feet have a chance to build up strength to support the additional work you are asking

16 Heel that Pain, 2018. "How to Correct Posture from the Feet Up." Accessed December 9, 2019. https://heelthatpain.com/correct-foot-posture/

17 www.Lommell.com, 2019. "Proprioception, Alignment, Performance, and Foot Levelers: A Winning Formula." Accessed December 10, 2019. http://www.lommell.com/new_page_123.htm

of them. Going directly from a highly supportive shoe to a minimal shoe may be too much for the muscles in your feet all at once.

Lower leg (shin/calf)
The muscles in your lower leg primarily work to move your ankle and foot. Your calf is actually made up of two muscles. The soleus muscle sits underneath the gastrocnemius, and together, they're responsible for pointing your toes (or plantarflexion). When speaking about anatomical direction, "plantar" refers to the bottom, and "dorsi" (think dorsal fin on a dolphin) refers to the top.

The muscles on the front of your shin work to lift the ball of your foot off the ground or "dorsiflex" your foot. When you want to tap your foot, you are using your shin muscles to lift your foot.

Just behind the knee, the popliteus muscle is responsible for unlocking your knees while walking and acts when sitting down or standing up. It is the only muscle in the lower leg that acts only on the knee and does not affect the ankle.

Upper leg (thigh)
Your thigh muscles are the primary group that acts on the knee. The front of your thigh is made up of the quadricep group, four muscles that work to extend (straighten) your knee. These are the rectus femoris, vastus lateralis, vastus medialis, and vastus intermedius. The rectus femoris also connects through to your hip and serves as one of the hip flexor muscles.

The back of your thighs is known as the hamstrings, a group of three muscles that flex (bend) the knee. These are the bicep femoris, semimembranosus, and semitendinosus.

Your inner thigh has its own group of five muscles that work to bring your legs together, and these are referred to as the adductor muscles.

Your outer thigh muscles work to lift the leg away from the body's midline and are referred to as the abductors. Sometimes you might hear your health care professional say "A-B ductors" because it is hard to hear the distinction between "abductors" and "adductors."

Hips and Buttocks Muscles

Your hips have the largest muscle in your body as one of your butt muscles: the gluteus maximus. Its role is to extend and externally rotate the hip joint and to keep the trunk of your body in an erect posture.

But your butt (I just had to say that) has two more often-overlooked muscles that are responsible for side leg lift (also considered part of your A-B ductor group). The gluteus minimus and gluteus medius help with how you place your leg in space. These muscles are under the gluteus maximus. If these muscles are weak, you'll sometimes see knees caving in when doing a squat.

There are many other smaller muscles that work to move the hip joint and thigh by connecting your pelvis to your femur.

Your hip flexor muscles help you lift your thigh and flex or hinge at the hip.

Core Muscles

The muscles of the abdomen and low back, which are primarily responsible for stabilizing the pelvis, are commonly known as core muscles. Your core muscles influence spine, hip, and rib cage position, which is vital for a stable trunk position. They include and are underneath many of the showier "six-pack" ab muscles.

If your core muscles are weak, your body may recruit your hip flexors to help stabilize your pelvis, which can cause your pelvis to rotate, which creates a chain reaction to your hamstrings.

Now that we have a basic understanding of how the knee and leg work together, let's move on to the exercises you need to strengthen the whole system.

CHAPTER 5

HEALTHY KNEES STRENGTH SOLUTION: YOUR PLAN & THE EXERCISES

As with any exercise program, please seek your doctor's approval before starting this one.

For each exercise, we list the purpose of the activity and the how-to instructions for completing the move.

In the world of strength training, there are many, many paths to the destination. While we have not included every single exercise possible (that would be overwhelming!), we narrowed it down to the essential moves to help your knees start feeling better.

We start at the basics and want you to master each move before moving on to the next. Now, with that said, you may have some discomfort because you haven't asked your body to move in this way before. It is important to know that no training program is without its ups and downs. As you train, you may be using your muscles in a different way, and you may feel some muscle soreness or joint achiness. A major part of overcoming discomfort is learning to recognize it, manage it, and work around it. We want you to be able to distinguish between pain (such as a sharp warning sign to stop) and discomfort (an ache or soreness). We seek to train in a pain-free manner and do not want to exacerbate any current symptoms.

At the same time, like Jillian Michaels tells her clients, *"get comfortable with being uncomfortable."*

We want you to learn to find a comfortable range of discomfort to work within. Something that you feel okay with and that does not last for too long after performing the exercise. If we train one day and you are muscle-sore or even a little achy joint sore the next day or two, that is often a sign that your body is adapting and getting stronger. Do not let it discourage you, as the discomfort should diminish with time. It's generally okay to keep exercising when you are sore, just make sure to give your body time to recover (a day off in between workouts), stay hydrated, and get plenty of sleep.

EQUIPMENT

Many of the exercises are bodyweight only, though some advance to using a piece of equipment that assists in muscle development. A list of the equipment we mention in this section is provided below. If you belong to a fitness club, this equipment will likely be available there. If you are doing these exercises at home, there are often substitutes you can make from items around your home.

To make it a little easier for you, we have put together a kit with the equipment shown below. You can purchase this kit from HealthyKneesCoach.com/shop.

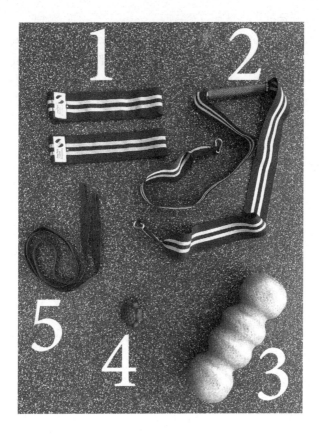

1. **Mini-band**—This is a small circular band that can stretch to
    about two times its length. It comes in a variety of materials.
    Our favorite is the wider elastic band shown in the picture
    (from Anchor Point Training) because it will not curl up
    as you put it on. The bands often come in sizes or different
    levels of resistance.

2. **Suspension Strap**—This is a thick elastic band with hooks
    on each end and a handle that slides to adjust along the
    strap. The band attaches to a door strap (#5 in the picture),
    which keeps it secure. The "anchor point" refers to where

the Suspension Strap is attached to the door. Directions for using the suspension strap usually call for "facing the anchor point" (meaning the front of your body is facing the point where the Suspension Strap is fastened to the door) or "facing away from the anchor point" (meaning the back of your body is facing the anchor point).

3. **Foam Roller**—This is usually a long cylinder of 4-6-inch diameter, made of a dense molded poly material. It comes in a variety of lengths from about 18 inches to 48 inches. The Rollga foam roller shown here is "shaped" for more support to your muscles as you roll.

4. **Helo Massage Ball**—The Rollga Helo Massage Ball uses neuro activators (rough bumps designed to grab skin) on one side and a round lacrosse ball feature on the opposite side to both stimulate fascia and unlock tension and stress. Additionally, tiny nodes or 'fingers' fill the circumference of the ball designed to pinpoint trigger points and address fascial scaring. The Helo Massage Ball takes the premise of a lacrosse ball and adds three more recovery friendly applications. We use this ball for the Piriformis Release.

5. **Door Strap**—This strap allows you to connect the Suspension Strap to any standard door. Not pictured:

   • Dumbbell—This is a short bar with a weight at each end and comes in a variety of weight denominations. If you don't have dumbbells at home, you can hold anything heavy to create the extra resistance. You can also use a weighted ball for many of the exercises

- Chair, Plyobox, Weight Bench—We do "sit-to-stand" exercises, and so you'll need something to sit on! If a chair or weight bench seems too low, try using a higher Plyobox at your fitness club, or a sturdy tabletop or your bed at home.

- Rolled Up Towel (for stretching assists and quadricep engagement exercises)

- Foam Pad—This is a thick square of foam to give some cushion to your knees when kneeling or can be used for standing balance challenges.

HEALTHY KNEES BUILDING BLOCKS: THE 4 POINT METHOD

Strengthening your knees involves more than just pushing weights and working on the muscles attached only to your knees. Our Four Point Method provides you with the building blocks for strong, healthy knees and legs.

1. Movement Foundations
2. Balance Training
3. Strength Training
4. Stretch Techniques

The list of exercises is grouped by the four building blocks. The 8-week plan mixes the exercises into the correct flow and advancement for you. The exercise descriptions that follow the plan are presented in the order you'll find them in the plan.

Many of the building block moves offer variations and advancements.

MOVEMENT FOUNDATIONS

In our Movement Foundations, we start with the essential movement elements that are the foundation for everything else. Our bodies are smart. We've said this a few times in this book. Movement Foundations is also where we outsmart our bodies. What I really mean is that we are going to work to break apart compensating actions and hopefully break bad habits.

There are seven Movement Foundations:

1. Short Foot
2. Pelvic Tilts
3. Abdominal Bracing
4. Belly Breathing
5. Glute Pops and Quad Squeezes
6. Knee Knockouts
7. Elements of the Squat

BALANCE TRAINING

Working on your body's ability to balance will help you prevent falls, correct for some compensations, and improve your kinesthetic awareness or ability to know where your body is in three-dimensional space.

A long time ago, I was given a very useful tip: if you find balance is a challenge, press your hands together in front of you or touch your body (like hips and shoulders) with your hands. This helps your proprioceptive nerves understand where your body is to create balance.

Balance Training is something you can do, even when you are waiting in line. Just stand on one foot! The more you practice, the better you'll get. All balance moves should be done on each leg, even if one is weaker than the other. Your body needs the training both ways.

We have four essential balance training moves for you:

1. Tandem Balance
2. Single Leg
3. Tree Pose
4. "T" Pose

STRENGTH TRAINING

Muscle development is part of gaining strength, building stamina, and creating freedom of movement. Don't worry, you are not going to get "bulky" from these exercises, but you may notice that with time, you have nicer muscle definition. We've divided the strength training exercises into four predominant areas that must be strengthened to have healthy knees.

Strength Training—Knee Dominant

These exercises directly work the muscles affecting the knee joint. Some moves have multiple variations and progressions that you will see in the exercise descriptions.

There are four main Knee Dominant moves:

1. Terminal Knee Extension
2. Sit to Stand
3. Goblet Squat
4. Step Ups and Step Downs

Strength Training: Hip Dominant
The exercises that directly affect the hip also act on the pelvis and thigh bone (femur). Since the femur is also part of your knee joint, what happens at the hip affects the knee. There are four main hip dominant exercises, each with variations:

1. Hip Hinge
2. Glute Bridge
3. Side Leg Lift
4. Deadlift

Strength Training: Ankle and Calf
Your calf muscles help bend your knees and lift the heel and point your toes (plantar flexion). The fronts of your shins help control the lift of the top of your foot (dorsi flexion). Strengthening your lower leg muscles will help give you more control of leg movement, and that is good for your knees!

We focus on one main ankle and calf strengthening move and offer many variations.

1. Standing Heel Raise (& variations)

Strength Training: Core
Strengthening your core muscles is important for stabilization of your hips and spine.

There are thousands of core strengthening moves. We selected a few that can be done standing and others that require getting on hands and knees on the floor. If knees on the floor is a challenge for you, try kneeling on a foam pad to give a little more cushion and support.

There are three main core moves with variations and advancements:

1. Pallof Press
2. Suitcase Holds
3. Bird Dogs

STRETCH TECHNIQUES
Regular stretching helps prepare your muscles for the work to come and improves flexibility and range of motion in your joints. Stretches should be done on each leg.

We have divided the stretches into three groups.

1. Dynamic Stretches
2. Static Stretches
3. Release Techniques

Dynamic Stretches
Dynamic stretching means you are moving through the stretch positions. It is a great way to prepare your muscles for the activity ahead. We use it to warm up your hips and knees.

1. Quadruped Rocking and Hold
2. Pigeon Rocking
3. Hip Hurdles

Static Stretches

Static Stretching means you hold the stretch position. To have the best results, static stretching should be done after you have warmed up or post exercise. We suggest holding each stretch from 30 seconds to two minutes.

1. Calf
2. Hamstring
3. Side Leg Stretch
4. Figure 4 Hip
5. Quadriceps
6. Half-Kneeling Hip Flexor

Release Techniques

The current literature measuring the effects of self-myofascial release is still emerging. Fascia is a web of connective tissue that covers every internal structure of the body. We've included foam rolling in this book because I've personally had so much relief from performing regular rolling on my own legs. It is definitely worth a try and, with time, if it makes you feel better, great! The trigger point method places pressure on a sensitive or sore spot in a muscle so that when the pressure is released, the muscle relaxes. Foam rolling and trigger point can be done either pre- or post-exercise.

1. Trigger Point
2. Foam Rolling

YOUR HEALTHY KNEES 8-WEEK PLAN

How to read the plan:

We advise you to do the exercises in the order presented in the plan. We have explained the reason and flow to the work, starting with warming up and balance challenges and working toward the bigger muscle groups.

The exercise descriptions that follow the plan are in the same order as you see them in the plan. On some weeks we will introduce new exercises to exchange for others.

When you see something like "10x," it means to complete the move ten times.

When you see something like "2x10," it means to complete two sets of ten repetitions. Either take a break between the sets or do a different exercise in between.

"RIR" means "repetitions in reserve," meaning that you have a little more you could do, but don't go there. You want to feel that your muscle is tired, but not have muscle failure to complete a repetition. If you see "3x3 RIR," it means to do three sets of as many repetitions as you can but stop when you think you could only do three more.

How do you know when you have 3 RIR? This is based on your perceived exertion and muscle fatigue. If you really aren't sure, try doing three more and see how you feel. If it is absolutely ALL you can do, then you have judged correctly. If you CAN do the three more and still feel like you have even more you could do, you can adjust your repetitions or add more weight.

We often say to stand with feet "hip-width apart" or "shoulder width" apart. This is truly a matter of comfort. If you feel like a narrower or a slightly wider stance feels better, do it! You can decide, based on comfort if your toes are pointed straight ahead or turned slightly out.

When you see "ea." It means to repeat the exercise on each leg or each foot.

Doing the exercises:
Although proper form is important, it is unrealistic to believe you will move with 100% correct form at first, or all the time for that matter. Do not be worried if your form is a little off at first, but rather, focus on moving slowly and intentionally with a weight you know you can control. Then, work toward better execution as you move forward week to week. The risk of injury is increased if you try to make large jumps in weight too quickly or try to go too fast. Make small changes week to week, rather than large jumps in one session.

When using dumbbells, kettlebells, or other weights, a good rule of thumb is to add no more than 10% if you are going to lift a heavier weight. When you go up in weight, it's okay to then reduce the number of repetitions if you need to. If you aren't ready to lift the next heaviest weight, you can add in a few more repetitions at your current weight.

This set of exercises will take about 45 minutes per exercise session. We'd like you to repeat the workout 2 or 3 times in the week, giving a day of rest in between.

You'll notice that some of the exercises drop off the weekly list as others are introduced. You can keep on doing all of the exercises if you have time. Some movements have variations. When variations are offered, start with the least challenging and choose an advancement when you have mastered the first movement.

HEALTHY KNEES STRENGTH PLAN: WEEKS 1 & 2

MOVEMENT FOUNDATIONS
Short Foot – 5x ea.
Pelvic Tilts -10x
Abdominal Bracing – 5x
Belly Breathing – 5x
Glute Pops – 5x & Quad Squeeze – 5x
Knee Knockouts – 5x
Elements of the Squat – 2x

STRETCH TECHNIQUES: DYNAMIC
Quadruped Rocking – 10x
Pigeon Rocking – 10x
Hip Hurdles – 5x ea.

STRENGTH TRAINING: CORE/HIPS
Glute Bridge – 2x10
Bird Dogs – 2x10

BALANCE TRAINING
Tandem Balance – 2x30 sec

MOVEMENT FOUNDATIONS
Weight Shifts w/MB @ Knee/Ankle – 2x10 repetitions (add mini-band if possible)

STRENGTH TRAINING: KNEE DOMINANT
Terminal Knee Extension – 2x10 Left/Right
Sit to Stand – 2x5

STRENGTH TRAINING: HIP DOMINANT
Hip Hinge – 2x10

STRENGTH TRAINING: CORE
Pallof Press – 2x10

STRENGTH TRAINING: CALF/ANKLE
Standing Heel Raise—2x10

STRETCHES: STATIC—hold 30 sec.-2 min.
Calf
Hamstring
Side Leg stretch
Hip
Quadriceps

STRETCH TECHNIQUES: RELEASE
Piriformis Release

HEALTHY KNEES STRENGTH PLAN: WEEK 3

MOVEMENT FOUNDATIONS
Short Foot – 5x ea.
Pelvic Tilts – 10x
Abdominal Bracing – 5x
Belly Breathing – 5x
Glute Pops – 5x & Quad Squeeze – 5x
Knee Knockouts – 5x
Elements of the Squat – 2x

STRETCHES: DYNAMIC
Quadruped Rocking – 10x
Pigeon Rocking – 10x
Hip Hurdles – 5x ea.

STRENGTH TRAINING: CORE/HIPS
Glute Bridge – 2x15
Bird Dogs – 2x15

BALANCE TRAINING
Tandem Balance – 2x30 sec

MOVEMENT FOUNDATIONS
Weight Shifts w/mini-band @ Knee/Ankle – 2x10 w/ band if possible
Single-Leg Toe Taps – 2x5 ea. with mini-band if possible

STRENGTH TRAINING: KNEE DOMINANT
Terminal Knee Extension – 2x12 ea.
Sit to Stand – 3x5
Elevate heels if needed
w/ or w/o band
Add counterbalance for assistance
Suspension Strap assist if needed

STRENGTH TRAINING: HIP DOMINANT
Hip Hinge – 2x10
Side Leg Lift – 2x10 ea.

STRENGTH TRAINING: CORE
Pallof Press – 2x12 with 5-second hold

STRENGTH TRAINING: CALF/ANKLE
Standing Heel Raise – 2x10 Hold dumbbells if ready

STRETCHES: STATIC—hold 30 sec.-2 min.
Calf
Hamstring
Side Leg stretch
Hip
Quadriceps

STRETCH TECHNIQUES: RELEASE
Piriformis Release

HEALTHY KNEES STRENGTH PLAN: WEEK 4

MOVEMENT FOUNDATIONS
Short Foot – 5x ea.
Pelvic Tilts – 10x
Abdominal Bracing – 5x
Belly Breathing – 5x
Glute Pops- 5x & Quad Squeeze – 5x
Knee Knockouts – 5x
Elements of the Squat – 2x

STRETCHES: DYNAMIC
Quadruped Rocking – 10x – add 30 sec. hold on last one
Pigeon Rocking – 10x
Hip Hurdles – 5x ea.

BALANCE TRAINING
Single-Leg Balance – 2x15-30 sec. ea.

MOVEMENT FOUNDATIONS
Single-Leg Toe Taps – 2x10 ea. with mini-band if possible

STRENGTH TRAINING: KNEE DOMINANT
Terminal Knee Extension – 2x15 ea.
Sit to Stand – 3x4
Elevate heels if needed
w/ or w/o band
Add counterbalance for assistance
Suspension Strap Assist if needed

STRENGTH TRAINING: HIP DOMINANT
Side Leg Lift or Clamshell 2x10 ea.

Deadlift – 3x5

STRENGTH TRAINING: CORE
Pallof Press – 2x12 add J-Hook

STRENGTH TRAINING: CALF/ANKLE
Standing Heel Raise w/variation – 2x10

STRENGTH TRAINING: CORE/HIPS
Glute Bridge – 2x15
Bird Dogs – 2x15

STRETCHES: STATIC—hold 30 sec.-2 min.
Calf
Hamstring
Side Leg stretch
Hip
Quadriceps

STRETCH TECHNIQUES: RELEASE
Piriformis Release

HEALTHY KNEES STRENGTH PLAN: WEEK 5 - DELOAD

STRETCH TECHNIQUES: DYNAMIC
Quadruped Rocking—10x – add 30 sec. stretch
Pigeon Rocking – 10x
Hip Hurdles – 5x ea.

BALANCE TRAINING
Single-Leg Balance – 2x15-30 sec. ea.
MOVEMENT FOUNDATIONS
Single-Leg Toe Taps – 2x5 ea. with mini-band if possible

STRENGTH TRAINING: KNEE DOMINANT
Sit to Stand – 2x5
Elevate heels if needed
w/ or w/o band
Add counterbalance for assistance
Suspension Strap Assist if needed

STRENGTH TRAINING: HIP DOMINANT
Side Leg Lift or Clamshells – 2x10 ea.
Deadlift – 2x3

STRENGTH TRAINING: CORE
Pallof Press – 1x12

STRENGTH TRAINING: CALF/ANKLE
Standing Heel Raise w/variation 1x10

STRETCH TECHNIQUES: RELEASE
Foam Roll (quads, side leg)

STRETCHES: STATIC—hold 30 sec.-2 min.
Calf
Hamstring
Side Leg stretch
Hip
Quadriceps
½ Kneeling Hip Flexor Stretch – 30 sec

STRETCH TECHNIQUES: RELEASE
Piriformis Release

HEALTHY KNEES STRENGTH PLAN: WEEK 6

STRETCH TECHNIQUES: DYNAMIC
Quadruped Rocking – 10x – add hold 30 sec.

Pigeon Rocking – 10x

BALANCE TRAINING
Single-Leg Balance – 2x30 sec. each. Optional Tree Pose

MOVEMENT FOUNDATIONS
Single-Leg Toe Taps – 2x15 ea.

STRENGTH TRAINING: KNEE DOMINANT
Goblet Squat – 3x3 RIR

Sit to Stand (if no gob. squat) – 3x3 RIR

Step-ups – 10x ea.

Step-downs – 10x ea.

STRENGTH TRAINING: HIP DOMINANT
Clamshells – 2x10 ea.

Deadlift – 3x5

Y Balance (start with the reverse portions, only add front if feels good)

STRENGTH TRAINING: CORE
Suitcase Hold – 2x20 sec

Pallof Press – 2x12 – Try narrow foot stance

STRENGTH TRAINING: CALF/ANKLE
Standing Heel Raise w/variation – 2x3

STRENGTH TRAINING: CORE/HIPS
Glute Bridge – 2x15 – try marching
Bird Dogs – 2x15—try adding elbow to knee crunch between extensions

STRETCH TECHNIQUES: RELEASE
Foam Roll (quads, side leg)

STRETCHES: STATIC—hold 30 sec.-2 min.
Calf
Hamstring
Side Leg stretch
Hip
Quadriceps
½ Kneeling Hip Flexor Stretch

STRETCH TECHNIQUES: RELEASE
Piriformis Release

HEALTHY KNEES STRENGTH PLAN: WEEK 7

STRETCH TECHNIQUES: DYNAMIC
Quadruped Rocking – 10x add hold 30 sec.

Pigeon Rocking – 10x

BALANCE TRAINING
Single-Leg Balance – 2x30 sec. each—try Tree Pose

MOVEMENT FOUNDATIONS
Single-Leg Toe Taps – 2x15 ea. with mini-band if possible

STRENGTH TRAINING: KNEE DOMINANT
Goblet Squat – 3x3 RIR or

Sit to Stand (if no gob. squat) – 3x3 RIR

Step-ups – 10x ea.

Step-downs – 10x ea.

STRENGTH TRAINING: HIP DOMINANT
Clamshells or Side Steps with Mini-band – 10x ea.

Deadlift – 4x6

Y Balance 5x ea. (start with the reverse portions, only add front if feels good)

STRENGTH TRAINING: CORE
Suitcase Hold – 2x20 sec

Pallof Press – 2x12 Try staggered step (lunge step)

STRENGTH TRAINING: CALF/ANKLE
Standing Heel Raise w/variation – 2x3 RIR

STRENGTH TRAINING: CORE/HIPS
Glute Bridge – 2x15—try marching
Bird Dogs – 2x15 add crunch or try Bear Hold

STRETCH TECHNIQUES: RELEASE
Foam Roll (quads, side leg)

STRETCHES: STATIC—hold 30 sec.-2 min.
Calf
Hamstring
Side Leg stretch
Hip
Quadriceps
½ Kneeling Hip Flexor Stretch

STRETCH TECHNIQUES: RELEASE
Piriformis Release

HEALTHY KNEES STRENGTH PLAN: WEEK 8

STRETCH TECHNIQUES: DYNAMIC
Quadruped Rocking – 10x add hold 30 sec.

Pigeon Rocking – 10x

BALANCE TRAINING
Single-Leg Balance – 2x30 sec. each or Tree pose or "T" pose

MOVEMENT FOUNDATIONS
Single-Leg Toe Taps – 2x15 ea. with mini-bands if possible

STRENGTH TRAINING: KNEE DOMINANT
Goblet Squat – 4x3 RIR or

Sit to Stand (if no gob. squat) – 3x3 RIR

Step-ups – 10x ea.

Step-downs – 10x ea.

STRENGTH TRAINING: HIP DOMINANT
Clamshells or Side Steps with Mini-band 10x ea.

Deadlift – 4x6

Y Balance – 5x ea.

STRENGTH TRAINING: CORE
Suitcase Hold – 2x20 sec

Pallof Press – 2x12—try holding press as you step away from anchor point

STRENGTH TRAINING: CALF/ANKLE
Standing Heel Raise w/variation – 2x3 RIR

STRENGTH TRAINING: CORE/HIPS
Glute Bridge – 2x15 try marching or single leg
Bird Dogs or Bear Holds- 2x15

STRETCH TECHNIQUES: RELEASE
Piriformis Release
Foam Roll (quads, side leg)

STRETCHES: STATIC—hold 30 sec.-2 min.
Calf
Hamstring
Side Leg stretch
Figure 4 Hip
Quadriceps
Half-Kneeling Hip Flexor

EXERCISE DESCRIPTIONS

For an easy-to-use printable guide with pictures of every exercise, go to www.healthykneescoach.com/HKStrength

Week 1 & 2 Exercise Descriptions

Don't Panic! There are a ton of exercises introduced this week because you are just starting out. This first week may take you extra time. Pretty soon, these exercises will become familiar, and you will feel like a pro.

MOVEMENT F OUNDATIONS

Short Foot   **Weeks 1-4**

Purpose: Short Foot exercises are used to strengthen the foot muscles (especially the arch) and improve your balance.[18] If the arch of your foot collapses, it follows that your knees may become knock-kneed (or valgus).

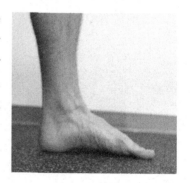

How To: Best done barefoot, while seated or standing. Grip the floor with your toes and lift up with your arch, like you are trying to suction your foot to the floor. If you look at your bare foot while doing this, you'll see your foot actually gets a little shorter (thus the name).

---

18   US National Library of Medicine, National Institutes of Health, 2019. "Short-Foot Exercise Promotes Quantitative Somatosensory Function in Ankle Instability: A Randomized Controlled Trial." Accessed December 18, 2019. https://www.ncbi.nlm.nih. gov/pmc/articles/PMC6350454/

It is not a big movement but will work to strengthen foot muscles, improve leg alignment, and improve balance.

Pelvic Tilts   Weeks 1-4

Purpose: Pelvic tilts serve as a good educational exercise to allow you to better feel your abdominals and their actions. This will allow you to better utilize them during exercise. This exercise also helps to correct for anterior pelvic tilt where the hip flexors are shortened, and hip extensors are lengthened, causing an excessive curvature of the low back.

How To (Standing): Stand with your feet hip-distance apart and relax your spine. Place your hands on your hips and rock your pelvis to create more of an arch in your low back, then rock your pelvis the opposite way to thrust your hips forward and create less of an arch in your low back.

How To (Lying on the Floor): Lying face up with your knees bent and your feet flat on the floor, place your hands under your low back. Using your hips and abdominals, press your low back into your hands or the floor. You'll feel like you are rotating your pelvis. Now release the pressure and create a small arch in your back by pressing your pelvis down toward your butt.

Abdominal Bracing   Weeks 1- 4

Purpose: We want to help you understand where your core muscles are located, so you have better control later on. Abdominal bracing is all about contracting your core muscles like you are bracing yourself against someone who is going to tickle you! As you do this, you create a natural belt or girdle of muscle that protects you. The muscles involved are the transversus abdominis, the rectus abdominus, the internal and external obliques, the pelvic floor muscles, and the multifidus muscle.

How To: While standing with feet hip-width apart, squeeze or contract your belly as if someone is going to tickle you. At the same time, suck up the floor of your abdomen as if you are guarding (or pulling up) your private parts (the same feeling as doing a "Kegel").

Belly Breathing   Weeks 1-4

Purpose: Well, of course, we all need to breathe. But HOW we breathe makes a difference, especially during exercise. We want you to become aware of your breath and how you can breathe deeply rather than shallowly.

How to: Place your hands on your chest and take a breath in through your mouth, visualizing that you are breathing into your hands. Now, place your hands on your belly and take a deep breath through your nose and notice how your belly expands and the breath feels deeper than when you had your hands on your chest. Exhale through your mouth.

Next, keep your hands on your belly and try to replicate that deep breath while breathing through your mouth. We want to train your breathing to be nice and deep, no matter if you take in your breath through your nose or your mouth.

When you breathe through your nose, your olfactory nerves are stimulated to signal to your brain that oxygen is coming in, and you will naturally take a deeper breath. This is not true for mouth breathing and so training yourself to breathe deep will help during exercise—or even for stress relief.

Glute Pops and Quad Squeezes   Weeks 1-4
These two sound like they should be summer-time desserts, but alas, they are exercises (that you can do anytime)!

Purpose: Let's make sure you understand how to engage certain muscles: your gluteus maximus (butt) and quadricep (front of thigh) groups. With knee injuries or post-knee surgery, sometimes it's a little bit harder to "connect" with these muscles. We want to make sure you are in control.

How to (Glute Pops): Lie on your back with your legs straight. Now squeeze your butt (gluteus maximus), and you should feel your hips rise. Try squeezing only one side and then the other. If getting on and off the floor is a challenge, for now, you can do this one sitting in a chair.

How To (Quad Squeeze): Sitting on the floor, place a rolled-up towel or foam roller under one knee. Now squeeze your thigh (quadriceps), so your leg straightens. Repeat on other leg.

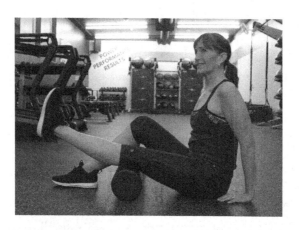

Knee Knockouts   Weeks 1-4

Purpose: Knee knockouts work on hip stability and gluteus minimus and medius (side butt muscles) strength.

How to: With a mini-band around your knees (can be at knees, above or below, find what is comfortable), assume a stance slightly wider than hip-width.

Try holding your foot stable on the floor and swing your knee to the side. If you do not feel the movement through your thigh and hip, try pivoting on the foot as if squashing a bug, slowly allow one knee to fall in towards the other, with the movement being produced from your hip. Then,

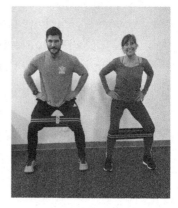

press the moving knee back out into the band, returning past the start position.

Elements of a Squat (hip hinge, knee bend)   Weeks 1-4

So many folks with knee issues fear squats, and I can understand why—because they can hurt! But they don't have to, and we hope to show you how best to squat for your body.

Purpose: Squats are a needed movement for everyday living. Learning to perform them properly, so you do not experience knee pain can be life-changing!

How to: We like to break down the squat into a flow of three pieces: Hip hinge, knee bend, open chest with a flat back. Start with your hands pressed together in front of you and your feet around hip

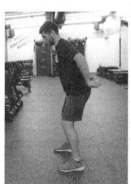 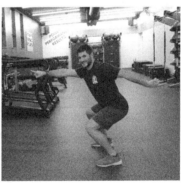

Hip break first, as hips go back, knees come forward (pointing for demonstration purposes only) shoulder-width apart. It is important to note that "feet hip-width apart" is just a societal "normal." It is a good starting position, but many people will require a wider or narrower squat stance to promote proper depth, comfort, and performance. Play around with the width of your feet and how pointed out your toes are to find the most comfortable position for you.

Feet can be pointing forward or slightly to the sides—whatever is more comfortable for you. Start with bending (hinging) at the hips first, then bending the knees to lower to the floor, while keeping the chest open with a flat back. Really push your booty out behind you! This avoids premature forward movement of the knee by shifting the hips backward.

Should your knees always stay behind your toes?

We believe it is a good rule of thumb that after bending at the hips, you allow your knees to move as far forward over your toes as comes naturally, while still maintaining balance and not overly provoking symptoms.

It is a common misbelief that your knees going out over your toes is a bad thing. This is a myth and adhering to it may cause more issues with the squat than allowing them to drift forward.

There comes a time when the lower leg (tibia) will begin to move forward in order to maintain balance. Your limb length will partially determine if or how far your knees may move forward over your toes. Trying to prevent knee movement over toes may result in you falling backward or putting too much strain on your hips and low back. Depending on the depth of your squat (and this has to do with the range of motion in your ankles and your knees), you may need your knees to clear your toes while squatting. Otherwise, you may have to compensate for the motion with excessive hip and low back movement. Allowing your knees to go over your toes as natural while you squat is a great way to load them, and to keep them strong and healthy.

Here are three "mistakes" to watch for (a mirror is handy here):

1. Do knees cave inward (valgus)?

As you descend in your squat, do you see your knees caving inward? If so, it may be a sign that your gluteus minimus and medius muscles are weak, or that you lack motor control within the squat. To correct, place a mini-band just below your knees and press out with your knees to keep tension on the band as you squat.

2. Do your heels lift as you squat?

This can be a sign that you need to work on mobility in your ankles. The ability for your ankle to dorsiflex, or for your knee to be able to drive far out past your toes, is vital to a proper squat. If your heels lift while you squat, first, adjust your stance—you may need to stand wider or turn your feet out more. Stretching your calves can also help with this. Focus on pushing through your heels as you descend and rise from the squat.

3. Is your back hunched while you squat?

If you find yourself looking at the ground while you are squatting, your back is probably hunched. Keep your eyes on the horizon as you squat to help your chest stay open and back flat.

STRETCH TECHNIQUES: DYNAMIC
Quadruped Rocking + Hold   Weeks: ALL
Purpose: This is a passive range-of-motion drill meant to help provide more low level and low impact knee flexion volume, to promote better knee flexion ranges, and to gradually address the fear and sensation of deep knee bends.

After warming up your knee joint with the rocking (described below), try holding the stretch for at least 30 seconds and up to 2 minutes at a time (as long as it doesn't cause pain).

How to (Standing): If kneeling simply isn't something you can do just yet, you can do this warm-up while standing. Place your foot on a chair and rock into the knee bend until you feel pressure but not pain.

How to (Kneeling): Starting on all fours, with padding under your knees if needed, slowly rock your hips back towards your heels as far as possible, while staying within a tolerable level of discomfort (if there is any present with this movement). Try to keep your hips reaching back evenly, avoiding sitting farther back into one hip compared to the other. Hold for a second at the deepest part of the movement, then rock back forward and repeat.

Pigeon Rocking   Weeks: ALL
Purpose: This is a mobility drill designed to target the entire hip and its associated musculature, as well as the hip capsule itself. The goal is to open up both internal and external rotation at the hip, allowing for easier movement with some of the strength exercises later in the workout.

How To: Starting on all fours, straighten one leg as far as you can straight behind you. Then, swivel the other leg under your body to somewhere between a 45- and 90-degree angle compared to your midline. From there, take the straight leg, and reach it across your body, so you are creating more tension in the bent leg hip. Slowly rock your weight backward and bend the straight leg knee to drop it to the floor. You should feel a stretch increase in the opposite hip. Slowly rock back and forth, bending and straightening the knee to allow you to sink deeper and deeper into the stretch.

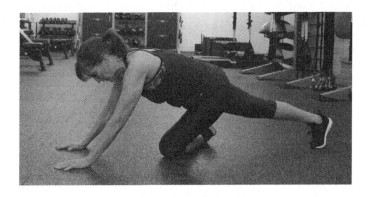

Hip Hurdles   Weeks 1-5
Purpose: To warm up your hip joint and work on mobility.

How To: Stand tall with your hands on your hips. Lift your right knee and leg up as if you are going to step over a fence or a hurdle. Rotate your knee to the right, keeping your leg high. Set your foot on the ground. Your feet should now make a 90-degree angle, with your left foot pointing forward and your right foot pointing to the right. Reverse the move by lifting your leg back up and over the imaginary hurdle. Place your foot back on the ground with both feet pointing forward. Repeat on left leg.

STRENGTH TRAINING: CORE/HIPS
Glute Bridge   Weeks 1-4, 6-8

Purpose: The Glute Bridge helps strengthen your posterior chain (backside) with emphasis on the big butt muscle (gluteus maximus) and back of thigh (hamstrings). It also serves to strengthen core muscles and can often alleviate low back pain.

How to (Standing Hip Extension Option): If the start position on the floor is a bit too difficult for you, stand erect, using support with hands on a wall or the back of a chair. Squeeze your butt and lift one leg slightly backward, keeping your knee straight. Be mindful to keep your hips stable and do not arch your back. You may only lift your foot about three to four inches off the floor.

If you are not sure you are doing this right, place one hand on your butt, and you should feel it tighten as you lift your leg behind you.

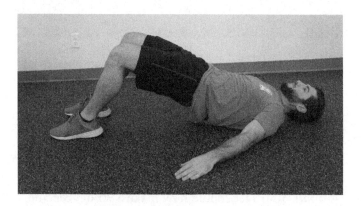

How to (Supine position): Lie face up on the floor (supine), with your knees bent and feet flat on floor with heels as close to your booty as you can. Place your hands on the floor, palms down next to your hips. Exhale, squeeze your butt, and lift your hips off the ground so that you form a straight line from knees to shoulders.

Work to hold the elevated position. Inhale as you return your hips to the ground.

If you notice that your knees dip together during the hip bridge, place a mini-band around both of your legs, just above your knees. Perform the exercise while keeping tension on the mini-band, not allowing it to go slack as you raise your hips.

Advance this Move—Marching in place: While in the bridge position and keeping hips high, "march" your feet, lifting one leg off the ground at a time. Try not to rock your hips or let them drop.

Advance this Move—Single Leg: When you feel stable with marching, try single-leg. In the starting position, squeeze your butt and lift one leg off the floor, pointing your foot at the ceiling. Drive your hips up into the bridge position, keeping your hips level to the floor. Return to start and repeat.

Bird Dogs   Weeks: 1-4, 6-7
Purpose: This move will help you improve core strength and balance.

How to (standing option): If getting onto hands and knees is not yet for you, try starting this move standing. Start with your hands on a wall at shoulder height, bearing some of your weight. As you step farther away from the wall, you'll place more weight on your hands. Keep your core tight and try to keep your body surfboard straight. As you slide one hand up the wall, lift the opposite leg behind you, keeping your leg straight and squeezing your butt. Only lift your leg as high as you can without arching your back. If you don't feel like you are doing this right, try poking yourself in the butt side of the lifting leg and making that muscle tense. Return to start and switch to other sides.

How to: Start in a tabletop position with hands and knees on floor with wrists directly under shoulders and knees under hips. Extend one arm without shifting your hips. Next, extend the opposite leg without shifting your hips. Once you've mastered this, lift and extend the opposite arm and leg at the same time without shifting your hips. Return to the tabletop start position, then switch to the other sides. The longer you hold the extension, the more challenging it is. This is definitely a balance move as much as a core move.

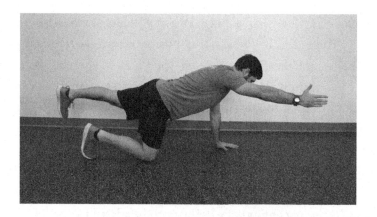

Advance this Move—Bird Dog with Crunch: When you are stable with both combos of arm and leg, try the bird dog with crunch. This can be done standing or in tabletop position.

How to (Bird Dog with Crunch): After you extend and reach your arm and leg, bring your knee and elbow together under your belly for a crunch. Tighten your abdominal muscles as you do this: pull your belly in like you are zipping up a tight pair of pants. For this version, do all the repetitions on one arm and leg combination, then switch to the other side.

Advance this Move—Bear Holds: The bear hold takes the bird-dog to the next level of challenge with a greater focus on core strength and balance.

How to (Bear Hold): Start on your hands and your knees in tabletop position. Round your back towards the ceiling, and then lift your knees 1-2 inches off the ground, hovering there for a 5-count (working up to 30 seconds) hold. During the hold, focus on taking slow breaths in through your nose, followed by forced exhales through your mouth. As you exhale, attempt to squeeze your abdominals tighter and tighter.

BALANCE TRAINING

Tandem Balance   Weeks 1-3

Purpose: The Tandem Balance takes your normal wide stance (feet under hips) and makes it narrow (feet in alignment with heel touching toe) in order to work on balance.

How to (with support): Stand near a wall and use one hand to gently support yourself as you get the feeling for this balance move. Place equal weight on each foot.

How to (without support): While standing, place one foot directly in alignment with the other with heel touching toe. Place equal weight on each foot. Then shift weight forward to put more weight on forward leg and shift weight backward to place more weight on back leg. Rock back and forth, pausing with balance on each leg.

How to (with head turning): Once you feel balanced without support, with your eyes open, try turning your head to look over your right shoulder, then over your left.

How to (with eyes closed): Go back to the corner for this. Align your feet, get balanced, then close your eyes, and maintain your balance.

How to (with movement): Right foot planted, move left foot in front, get balanced, then move left foot behind, get balanced. Change to your left foot planted with rotating your right foot in front and in back. Then keep advancing with several steps forward followed by several steps backward. When all of that feels pretty simple, rotate your head to look left and right as you step.

MOVEMENT FOUNDATIONS
Weight Shifts   Weeks 1-3
Purpose: We are beginning to work on a little balance here and waking up those gluteus minimus and medius muscles.

How to (without band): Standing upright with legs shoulder-width apart, slowly shift weight from one foot to the other as you rock side to side. You are not going to take one foot off the floor just yet. Rather, simply shift the majority of your weight from one foot to the other, rising to the ball of the non-weight-bearing foot.

How to (with band): Add a mini-band around your knees, mid shin, or ankle—the lower it is, the more challenging. The addition of the band will add resistance, and you will have to work to keep from allowing the band to pull your leg inward.

STRENGTH TRAINING: KNEE DOMINANT

Terminal Knee Extension   Weeks 1-4

Purpose: We want to get the attention of your quadricep muscles and make sure they are doing their job. This exercise is a good pre-cursor to the squat.

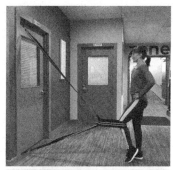

How to: Attach your mini-band through the Suspension Strap or around something solid like a table leg.

Step one leg inside the loop, bringing the band up to your knee. Stand far enough away from the table leg so that there is tension on the band. Allow the banded knee to bend as the band pulls it forward. Use control!

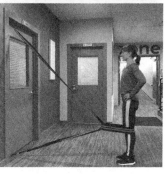

Then squeeze your quadricep muscles as you straighten your leg at the knee.

Sit to Stand   Weeks 1-4

Purpose: The Sit to Stand action is a basic life movement. We want you to feel strong and balanced, maybe even so strong that you don't have to push yourself up when you go to standing. We love the independence this strength brings. This move uses primarily your thigh and butt muscles.

There are four progressions of Sit to Stand to ultimately bring you to perform a squat. Start with #1 Wall Slides and work your way to #4 Sit to Stand with no weight. Remember, master your form before you move on to the next difficulty.

If you see that your knees are caving in as you squat, place a mini-band around both legs just above the knees and keep tension in the band throughout the movement.

Sit to Stand #1: Wall Slides

Wall slides begin to strengthen thigh muscles with the support of a wall so that you are not fully weight-bearing to your feet.

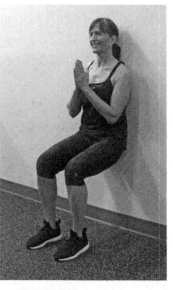

How to (Wall Slides): Start with leaning your back against a wall and feet about 2-foot lengths in front of the wall with knees are slightly bent. To perform the move, slide your back down the wall as you bend your knees until you come close to a "sitting" position. The goal is to bring your thighs parallel to the floor with a 90-degree bend in your knees, but it may take some practice before you can do this.

Adjust your feet so that your knees do not slide far in front of your toes. Hold the sitting position for 5 seconds then return to standing by sliding back up the wall to the start position. Work up to holding the sitting position for 60 seconds at a time. If your knees hurt during this move, try sliding down only as far as is comfortable, then push yourself back up.

This is an exercise favored by skiers to strengthen quad endurance.

Sit to Stand #2: Suspension Strap Squat

Suspension Strap Squat provides support from your arms holding on to the Suspension Strap. If you do not have access to a Suspension Strap, stay with the Wall Slide or move to the Sit to Stand with Counterbalance.

How to (Suspension Strap Squat starts with bent arms): While facing the anchor point of the Suspension Strap, grip the handles and place elbows at your side, creating tension on the Suspension Strap with a slight backward lean of your body (keep your body in a "surfboard straight" position from ankles to shoulders). Lower into the squat position while straightening your arms. You can use your arms to assist you in returning to a standing position. Go as low as feels comfortable. If you feel pain, stop just before that point. Conduct the Suspension Strap Squat and return to stand over 2-3 seconds each direction.

How to (Suspension Strap Squat with straight arms): For an added challenge while still assisted by the Suspension Strap, start in a standing position with arms straight and a slight lean backward. Lower into the squat position and return to standing while your arms are straight. This way, you are not using your arms as much to assist you in the return to standing. Conduct the Suspension Strap Squat and return to stand over 2-3 seconds each direction.

Sit to Stand #3: With Counterbalance

The assistance in this move comes from holding a weight at chest level and pressing that weight away from your chest as you sit.

This acts as a counterbalance to the weight of your hips as you hinge and press your booty back to sit.

How to: Start standing with your feet shoulder-width apart in front of the chair (or bench or Plyobox) you are going to sit on. Hold the weight at chest height and press the weight forward, keeping arms parallel to floor as you hinge your hips back and lower your booty toward the chair.

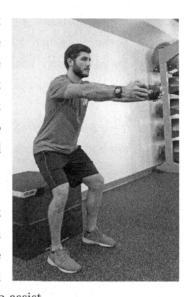

When you return to standing, start with the weight pressed out and then bring it back to your chest as you rise to stand. As you get stronger, you'll use a progressively lighter weight to assist.

Sit to Stand #4: No Weight
Once you feel like you have accomplished the Sit to Stand with a low weight, now it is time to try it with no weight.

How to: Start with holding your arms out in front if that helps to bring balance as you lower onto the seat and return to standing.

STRENGTH TRAINING: HIP DOMINANT

Hip Hinge   Weeks 1-3

Purpose: The hip hinge primarily targets your "backside" or posterior chain, with your glutes, hamstrings, and low back.

Start with the Suspension Strap supported Hip Hinge. If you do not have a Suspension Strap, move on to Hip Hinge #2 with Dowel.

Hip Hinge #1: Suspension Strap (supported)

Purpose: The Suspension Strap will give you support and let you feel the movement of pushing your hips back as you hinge forward.

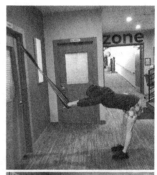

How to: With the Suspension Straps at mid-length, stand facing the anchor point with your arms straight and hands pressing down on the Suspension Strap handle. Feet are about shoulder-width apart. Inhale as you bend forward with a flat back, pushing your hips back and surfing your hands forward. To return to standing, exhale as you push your hips forward and keep the downward tension on the Suspension Strap handles.

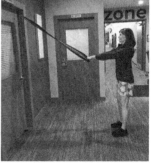

Hip Hinge #2: With Dowel

Purpose: Holding a dowel against your spine helps to prevent you from "cheating" by bending your back and releasing work from your hips and hamstrings.

How to: Use a broomstick or any sort of dowel to help force a flat back. Put the dowel behind you and hold it to your spine with one hand in the small of your back and one in the nape of your neck. Keep the dowel touching your head, middle back, and butt as you reach your hips backward and poke your chest out in front of you—picture pushing in a drawer with your hips, or boxing someone out in basketball.

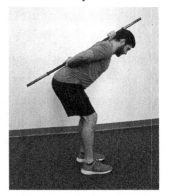

Hip Hinge #3: Good Morning

Purpose: This unsupported move prepares you for the deadlift and squat.

How to: Start standing with your feet shoulder-width apart and place your hands on your chest. Use good posture with shoulders back and brace your abdominals. Inhale as you hinge forward at your hips, pushing your booty behind. Have a slight bend in your knees. Try to create a 90-degree hinge, so your torso is parallel to the floor. Exhale as you return to standing.

Advance this Move: To make this move a little more challenging, change your center of gravity by placing your hands behind your head.

STRENGTH TRAINING: CORE

Pallof Press   Weeks: ALL

Purpose: The Pallof Press is an anti-rotation exercise that strengthens core muscles that help stabilize and protect your low back. The exercise was invented by physical therapist John Pallof.

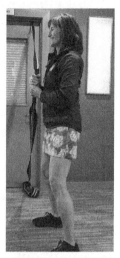

We love this exercise because you can do it standing, where many other core exercises require you to get on/off the floor.

How to: Use the Suspension Strap attached low and high and slide the handle to chest height to perform the Pallof Press. Hold the handle with both hands. Start side-facing to the attachment point in an athletic position (feet shoulder-width apart, slight bend in knees, chest up). Bring the handle to your chest, and there should be tension on the band.

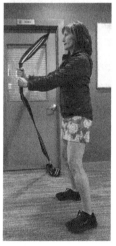

Exhale and press the handle straight forward. Resist the pull of the band toward the attachment; this is the "anti-rotation" part of the exercise. Return the handle to your chest. The slower you move, the harder it is.

Pallof Press Variations:
- Pallof Press with 5-second hold.
- Pallof Press with J-hook (Make a "J" movement when you are at straight arm press).
- Narrow your foot stance (bring feet closer together).
- Change feet to a lunge stance (one foot forward, one back).
- Pallof Press—walkout: as you are holding the press, take a step away from the anchor point, hold, and step back in.

STRENGTH TRAINING: CALF/ANKLE

Standing Heel Raise   Weeks: ALL

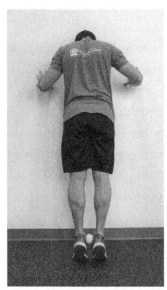

How to: Start out standing near a wall for balance. With your feet hip-width apart, lift your heels off the floor while pressing into the balls of both feet. Keep good posture with abdominal muscles pulled in so that as you lift your heels, your body shifts upward rather than forward or backward. This is one of our favorite moves to practice while standing in line at the grocery store.

Form tip: Place a tennis ball between your ankles to help your ankles to stay in line and not roll away from your mid-line.

Standing Heel Raise: with Weights
How to: Hold dumbbells at your side as you raise and lower your heels to increase the resistance and challenge. Keep increasing your weight as you get stronger. You can still use the tennis ball between your heels to ensure your ankles are not rolling out.

Standing Heel Raise: on Stair
How to: Standing with the balls of your feet on a stair, allow your heels to drop lower than the stair, then press up to the balls of your feet. Hold on to the stair rail or balance on the wall. Do this one slowly and with control as you stretch your Achilles Tendon with the heel drop.

Standing Heel Raise: Single Leg (supported)
How to: Using a wall for stability, balance on one leg, and raise your heel. When you feel confident, try this move without support.

STRETCH TECHNIQUES: STATIC
Calf Stretch   Week: ALL
Purpose: To help improve plantarflexion by stretching your calf muscles (located at the back of your shin).

How to: While standing, take a large step backward with one foot. With both feet pointing forward, keep your weight on your bent front leg. Bring the heel of your back leg toward the floor for a calf stretch with a straight leg. Take in a deep breath, raise your arms and eyes to the ceiling, exhale, and bring your arms back to your sides. Bring your feet together and repeat on the other side.

Hamstring Stretch Week: ALL

Purpose: To help improve range of motion through your hip by stretching your hamstring muscles (located at the back of your thigh).

How to: While standing, step one foot forward. Leave the forward heel on the ground, straighten your leg, and raise your toes. Transfer your weight to your back leg with knee slightly bent and a flat back. Hinge forward at your hips. Rest your hands on the tops of your thighs or, if you need help with balance, hold onto a chair. Take in a deep breath. As you exhale, stretch a little more and lift your toe even higher. Step back to standing and repeat on the other side.

Side Leg Stretch   Week: ALL

Purpose: This move helps stretch the muscles associated with the Iliotibial Band (ITB), which include your tensor fasciae latae and gluteus maximus muscles, both at your hip. The IT band itself is a very thick sheath of fascia (connective tissue) that runs the length of the outside of your leg from hip to knee. The ITB works to stabilize the hip during walking and acts as a spring to 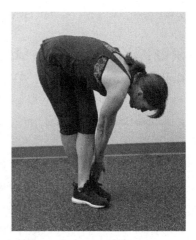 aid in running.[19] You may notice a difference in how far you can reach for on each side for this one.

---

19   The Harvard Gazette, 2015. "Understanding the IT Band." Accessed January 5, 2020. https://news.harvard.edu/gazette/story/2015/08/understanding-the-it-band/

How To: While standing cross your left foot in front of your right so that your feet are side-by-side. Now press your hands together. Hinge at your hips and reach with hands toward the instep of your back (right) foot. Hold, then return to standing. Complete the stretch on the other side.

Figure-Four Hip Stretch   Week: ALL
Purpose: To help improve range of motion in your hip by stretching the hip muscles. The figure-four stretch can be done standing or lying down. Do the one that feels the best for you and repeat on each leg.

How to (Standing Figure Four): Start with a slight bend in your knees and cross your left ankle over your right thigh, above your knee. To deepen the stretch, press on your left thigh (not your knee).

How to (Figure Four with Chair Assist): Shift your weight to your left leg and place right foot on a chair. Let the right knee and thigh press toward the floor. To deepen the stretch, press on your thigh (not your knee).

How to (Figure Four on the Floor): Lie with your back on the floor and cross your legs, bringing your knees toward your chest. Hug your knees, and you should feel a nice deep stretch in your butt. 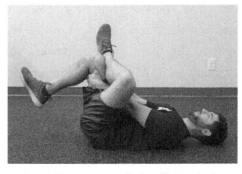 To deepen the stretch, press your shins toward the floor, as long as this does not irritate your knees.

How to (Figure-Four Reach Through): To make the floor stretch even deeper, cross your right ankle over your left thigh, just above your knee. Reach your right arm between your legs and clasp your left hand behind your left leg to gently pull your leg closer to your chest.

Quadriceps Stretch   Week: ALL

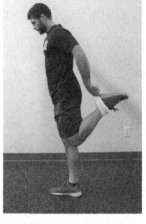

Purpose: To improve range of motion through your knee and hip by stretching the quadricep muscles (on the front of your thigh). The basic movement is to bend at the knee, bringing your heel toward your butt. Depending on your knee range of motion, you may need help with this one.

As you perform the stretch, keep your knees side by side and focus on standing tall with your hips pressed forward and shoulders back.

How to (Quad Stretch Assist with a Chair): Standing in front of a chair like you are going to sit down, raise one leg up behind you, and rest the top of your foot on the chair with your knee pointing toward the floor. You might want to be near a wall for balance and may need to bend the supporting leg to deepen the stretch.

How to (Quad Stretch Assist with a Towel): Start standing and bend over to wrap a small towel around one ankle. Hold the towel near your ankle with the same side hand. As you return to standing, lift your towel-ankle toward your butt behind you.

How to (No Assist Quad Stretch): This is only for you if you have the ability to fully flex your knee. If you have limited range of motion, use one of the assists.: While standing, bring your heel toward your butt and grab onto your ankle. Your knees should be side by side and body erect. If you go through any gymnastics to do this or your knee is sticking out to the side, or if you are side bending one way or the other, *don't!* This poor alignment could strain your back. Use one of the assists, above.

Half-Kneeling Hip Flexor Stretch   Week: ALL

Purpose: This passive stretch is designed to provide a stretch to the hip flexor (iliopsoas) muscle group and improve hip mobility.

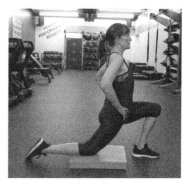

How To: Place the foam pad or a pillow beneath the right knee as you get into a half-kneeling position with your right knee down and left foot on floor in front of you. The left hip and leg should be flexed to 90 degrees. Next, fully raise your right arm overhead like you are trying to reach the ceiling. Squeeze your right butt (glute) and slowly shift your torso forward, allowing the right hip to extend. You should feel the stretch through the front of your right hip. To deepen the stretch, tuck your hips (posterior pelvic tilt).

STRETCH: TRIGGER POINT

Piriformis Release Week: ALL

The Piriformis is a muscle deep in your butt that originates at the sacrum (near your tail bone) and attaches to the side knob (greater trochanter) near the top of the femur. It helps to lift and rotate your leg away from the midline. The piriformis can irritate the nearby sciatic nerve and cause "Piriformis Syndrome" with pain originating in the buttocks and radiating down the leg. Of course, if you have sciatic nerve pain, please see your doctor! Sciatic pain can also be caused by compression in the spine.[20]

Purpose: I include this release because, to me, it feels good, and I feel like it helps my butt and my legs stay a little more relaxed. Does it actually help relax the muscle? I don't know, but you definitely feel the difference as soon as you complete the move.

How to: Use your Helo Massage Ball or use a hard ball, such as a lacrosse ball or tennis ball. While sitting on the floor with your legs extended straight in front of you, pretend you are slipping the ball into 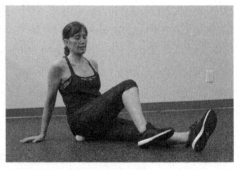 your back right pocket. Gently "sit" on the ball and position it on the spot that feels the most tender. Now bend and straighten your right leg four times, sliding your foot toward your butt, then back

---

20   National Academy of Sports Medicine, 2018. "Piriformis: Is it Really Tight? Really?" Accessed December 28, 2019. https://blog.nasm.org/fitness/piriformis-is-it-really-tight-really/

to straight leg. Next, with your right knee bent and foot on the ground, let your knee dip toward your left leg four times. Then, let your knee lower toward the floor away from your left leg, four times. Finally, straighten your leg, sit up tall, and—this is where the magic happens—remove the ball and feel the "cave" in your butt. NICE! Make sure to repeat this release on your left side.

WEEK 2 NEW EXERCISE DESCRIPTIONS

No new exercises! Keep it up!

WEEK 3 NEW EXERCISE DESCRIPTIONS

MOVEMENT FOUNDATIONS
Single-Leg Toe Taps   Weeks 3-8

Purpose: Working your abductor muscles (the muscles that help move your leg to the side and give your knees more stability.)

How to: Stand with a mini-band around both of your legs. Position the mini-band at your knees, mid-shin, or ankle (the lower it is around the leg, the more challenging). Stand with all of your weight balanced over one leg. With the other leg, reach at a 45-degree angle out to the side and backward, gently tapping your toe on the ground without placing any real weight through the moving foot. All of your body mass and weight should stay stacked over the standing leg, with the opposite limb moving against the tension of the mini-band.

STRENGTH TRAINING: HIP DOMINANT
Side Leg Lift   Weeks 3-5

Purpose: The Gluteus Medius and Minimus are two of the butt muscles that help stabilize the pelvis and are the prime movers and controllers for side leg movement.

Are you doing the moves, right? If you feel the work happening in your thigh (quadriceps), that means your toes are pointing up, and you need to point your toes toward the wall (not ceiling) or even toward the floor. You should definitely feel the work in your side butt, not on the front of your thigh.

How to (standing): Stand side facing to a wall with the closest hand for support, other hand on hip. With your knee straight and your toes pointed forward (not up!), exhale as you raise your leg to the side. Do not shift your hips as you do this exercise. Inhale as you return your leg to the start position.

How to (side lying on floor): Lie down on your side with legs extended and stacked, so your body is in a straight line. With toes pointed forward, exhale as you lift your top leg. Inhale as you return your leg to the stacked position.

WEEK 4 NEW EXERCISE DESCRIPTIONS

BALANCE TRAINING

Single-Leg Balance   Weeks 4- 8

Purpose: In order to further challenge your balance, we narrow your base of support to one leg, not two.

How to (starting with support): With your hand supported on a wall or a table or chair, shift your weight to the supporting leg and then lift the other foot off the ground. Try to reduce the amount of support you need so that you can balance while standing on just one leg.

How to (no support): Press your hands together in front of you, shift your weight to your supporting leg and lift one foot off the ground.

For one-minute, alternate standing single leg for 10 seconds per leg, then advance to 15 seconds per leg, 20 seconds, and so on until you can stand for one minute per leg without support.

How to (add a challenge and make it a habit): Practice standing on one leg while you brush your teeth. We love this move because we are tacking on a new habit to one you already have: brushing your teeth! Stand on one leg while you brush your lowers, then switch the other leg while you brush your uppers. This is an easy way to incorporate balance twice a day. The wiggling and jiggling while you brush helps to fine-tune your balancing muscles.

STRENGTH TRAINING: HIP DOMINANT

Clamshells   Weeks 4-8

Purpose: To strengthen hip abductor and external rotation muscles.

How to: Start lying on your side, with your legs together and knees bent so your heels are in line with your butt. Keeping your heels together, raise the knee of your top leg, so it points up toward the ceiling, then return to start. The slower you go, the harder it is.

Advance this Move: Place a mini-band around your thighs just above your knees for added resistance.

Deadlift   Weeks 4-8

Purpose: The deadlift directly targets all of the major muscle groups that are responsible for strong posture, core strength, and leg power. The primary muscle groups include gluteus maximus (butt), hamstrings (back of thigh), quadriceps (front of thigh), extensor spinae (low back), trapezius (upper back) and many other supporting muscles from your calves to core.

The key to success with the deadlift is to start with a lightweight so that you have the proper form before going to a heavier weight. You can use a kettlebell or single dumbbell held with both hands.

How to: Stand erect with your feet shoulder-width apart, with the weight on the floor between them. Deadlifts should be performed with the feet directly underneath the hips, but small adjustments can be made to accommodate the weight, as well as comfort. Bending at the waist, reach down and grab the weight. Before standing up, make sure to flatten your back and reach your hips back and slightly up to create tension in your hamstrings. The hips should be slightly higher than your bent knees.

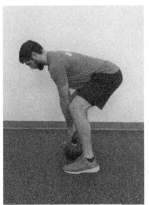 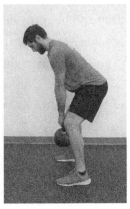 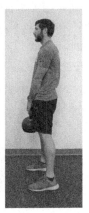

Your shoulder blades should be squeezed together and arms straight and close to your body (but not elbows locked) as you grab the weight. From here, take a deep breath in, squeezing your midsection tight, and push the floor away with your full foot. Slowly lift the chest keeping the arms straight. In doing so, the weight will slowly lift from the floor. Squeeze your butt tight at the top of the position

Advance this Move—Staggered Romanian Deadlift: This style of deadlift puts more work in your forward leg.

How to: Start standing and shift your weight to one leg (left) and take one step back with your right foot. Hold the weights in each hand with straight arms and keep them close to your body. As you hinge at the hips with slightly bent knees, lower the weights to about knee level then return to standing.

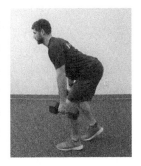

Advance this Move—Single-Leg Deadlift: The Single Leg Deadlift helps you to work on balance and single-leg strength.

How to: Start standing and holding weight with straight arms near your forward leg. Stagger your step and put your weight into your forward left leg. As you lift your right leg up, your torso will lean forward to create a "T" stance, and weight will point toward the floor and stay close to your shin as you lower and rise.

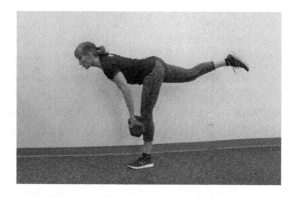

WEEK 5 NEW EXERCISE DESCRIPTIONS

De-load week! A little easier on your body. One new move meant to soothe sore or tired muscles.

STRETCHES: FOAM ROLLING

Foam Rolling   Weeks: 5-8

Foam rolling is possibly the best restorative technique I have ever used. At first, it can be painfully uncomfortable. As you consistently use a foam roller, you should find relief. Some studies have shown that foam rolling may be beneficial in relieving muscle soreness and improving passive and dynamic range of motion.[21] [22]

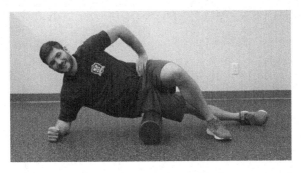

Foam rolling places a pressure (the roller) on your fascia and underlying muscle. I like to foam roll before I exercise when I am going to focus on range of motion; and after exercise, especially after long bike rides where my legs feel tired.

---

21 National Center for Biotechnology Information, 2019. *Frontiers in Physiology*, "A Meta-Analysis of the Effects of Foam Rolling on Performance and Recovery." Accessed January 5, 2020. https://www.ncbi.nlm.nih.gov/pmc/articles/PMC6465761/

22 Medicine and Science in Sports and Exercise, 2014. "Foam Rolling as a Recovery Tool After an Intense Bout of Physical Activity." Accessed January 5, 2020. https://journals.lww.com/acsm-msse/Fulltext/2014/01000/Foam_Rolling_as_a_Recovery_Tool_after_an_Intense.19.aspx.

Pay special attention to your quadriceps, Iliotibial band, hamstring, and calf. There are many techniques to rolling, but the one I find most beneficial is to lie on the roller and start just above your knee (never roll directly on the joint). Roll up about 4 inches, back 2 inches, up 4 inches, and back 2 inches, slowly inch-worming up your leg; then reverse direction and roll, using the same method back to your starting point.

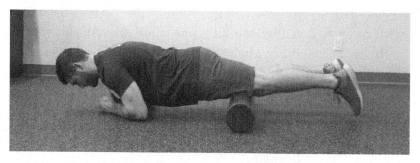

This does require a certain amount of core strength. If you are unable to maneuver your body onto the floor to use a foam roller, you can try sitting in a chair with your leg relaxed and use an old-fashioned rolling pin to roll your quads and IT band.

WEEK 6 NEW EXERCISE DESCRIPTIONS

STRENGTH: HIP DOMINANT

Y Balance   **Week: 6-8**

Purpose: We are incorporating balance and movement through the hip to improve strength and stability.

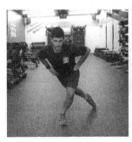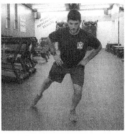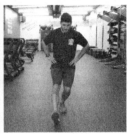

How to: Imagine there is an uppercase, upside-down "Y" on the floor. You will be standing on one leg, with your foot in the middle of the Y. Your goal is to keep all your weight and body mass over the standing leg. Both legs will have a slight bend at the knee. As you slide the foot of the opposite leg along each back portion of the Y, bend the knee and hinge at the hip of your supporting leg as your body lowers to reach as far as you can with your sliding foot. Return sliding foot to the middle and stand upright each time.

As you progress with the exercise, work on adding the "stem" of the Y by sliding your foot (heel) forward as you bend and load the supporting knee.

BALANCE

Tree Pose   Week 6-8

Purpose: To shift your center of gravity in order to challenge your ability to balance. Try this balance move only after you feel you are stable with the single-leg balance.

How to: With your hands pressed together in front of you, shift your weight to one leg. Then lift the other foot, and with your knee pointing out to the side, place your foot as high as you can on the inner side of your supporting leg—on your ankle, calf, knee, or thigh. Check your posture and stand up tall!

STRENGTH TRAINING: KNEE DOMINANT

Goblet Squat   Weeks 6-8

Purpose: The goblet squat works not only your legs and butt, but also arms, shoulders, and core as you hold and stabilize the weight.

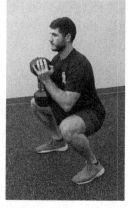

How to: Hold a dumbbell vertically with your hands, cupping the top end of the weight like you are holding a big goblet. Hold the weight at high chest level, with elbows pinned at your rib cage. Feet are about hip-width apart, with toes pointed forward or slightly out.

Keep your arms close to your chest and elbows pointing down. Bend your hips, then knees, to lower your body into a squat position as low as you can comfortably go over about 3 to 5 seconds. When you return to standing, drive through your glutes, legs, and heels to return to starting position, over about 3 to 5 seconds. Maintain control in both downward and upward movements.

Step Ups and Step Downs   Weeks 6-8

Purpose: Climbing stairs is an everyday activity, and we want you to be able to do this comfortably and with confidence. These moves build strength and control.

There are two variations for this exercise: Forward-Facing Step Up and Side-Facing Step Up to help strengthen and prepare you for stairs.

Forward-Facing   Step Up

How to: Start with a four-inch rise step. Most aerobics benches are about four inches without any risers. Most stair risers are six to seven inches high, which may be too high at the start. Place the foot of your working leg (right leg) on the stair, and as you bring the left foot up to the stair, think of pressing through your right hip as you step up. Then step your left foot back to the floor. Repeat on your right leg up to 15 times, then switch to the left.

Advance this Move: As you get stronger and 15 repetitions are no problem, advance to a higher rise or add holding a dumbbell in each hand. Keep on advancing as long as there is no pain.

Side-Facing   Step Downs

How to: Starting with a four-inch-high step, align your foot to the length of the step, so you are side-facing (if this was a stairway). Start with one foot on the step and one on the floor. Rise to a stair-standing position, pushing through the hips and straightening your knee. Bring your non-weight bearing leg level to the stair, but not on it. Then as you slowly lower, try to touch down with your heel or a flat foot, not your toe. This forces you to have more control over the weight-bearing leg on the stair.

Advance this Move: As you get stronger with this move, instead of landing with a flat foot, try just touching your heel to the floor, then return to stair standing position. Advance by increasing the step height or add holding a dumbbell in each hand.

CORE STRENGTH
Suitcase Holds   Weeks 6-8
Purpose: The suitcase hold is a basic but very functional exercise that strengthens core, shoulders, upper back, arms, and legs, as well as grip strength.

How to: Use a dumbbell or kettlebell or a heavy suitcase! Choose a weight that is heavy enough to create resistance, but not so heavy that it forces you to shift your posture. With feet shoulder-width apart, core muscles engaged, and shoulder blades pulled down and back, hold the object with one hand. Either simply hold the weight while standing in place or walk forward while maintaining good posture. Switch weight to the other hand, and repeat.

WEEK 7 NEW EXERCISE DESCRIPTIONS

Sidestep with Mini-band   Week 7-8
Basically, you are sidestepping in one direction while keeping tension on the mini-band. Then you will sidestep back to your starting point. Try 5-10 steps to start.

How to: Start with both legs inside the loop of one mini-band and place the mini-band at your knees. Assume the athletic stance (slight crouch) with feet wide enough apart to create tension on the mini-band. With your "lead" leg, take a step to the side, creating more tension with the mini-band, then bring your following leg toward it. Keep side-stepping in the same direction, take a break, then return to the athletic stance and sidestep your way back to your starting point.

Alternatives: To make this move easier, slide the band above your knees, or don't use a band at all. To make this move more challenging, place the band below your knees. This will create more lateral tension on your knee joint, which is good for strengthening. However, if it hurts, keep the band at or above your knees.

WEEK 8 NEW EXERCISE DESCRIPTIONS

BALANCE
"T" Pose   **Week 8**

Purpose: We use movement and a changing center of gravity to challenge your balance. Try this move after you feel stable with the single-leg balance and tree pose.

How to: Shift your weight to one leg. Imagine that you are a surfboard, from your shoulder to the foot of your non-weight bearing leg. Begin by starting the hinge at your hip, and as your torso hinges toward the floor and your hands pressed together reach forward in line with the "T," your non-weight bearing leg will lift up to keep surfboard straight from shoulder to ankle (or the best you can). Ultimately you are trying to form a "T" with your supporting leg as the base, and the two arms of the T as your lifted leg and leaning torso with arms extended.

CHAPTER 6

YOU HAVE MORE CONTROL THAN YOU THINK

WOW. You must be thinking that there are a whole lot of exercises involved with keeping your knees healthy and might be worried about actually getting going.

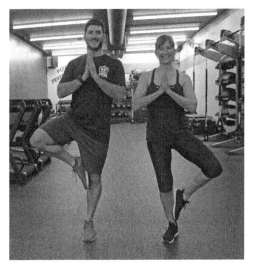

I want to now take the time to tackle some of your concerns about starting this strength training program for your knees. These are the concerns from our students who've been through our "live" Healthy Knees programs, and I thought it might be useful to you to hear the solutions.

THE 10 COMMON CONCERNS AND HOW TO RESOLVE THEM

1. I don't know where to start
Hopefully, we've solved that! It is exactly why we provided the information in this book—to give you the place to start. We break down the moves into the basic elements so you can master those first and feel confident before you are challenged with something more.

Starting your program will be fun! It's even a great excuse to go get yourself a new pair of athletic shoes and a comfy workout outfit.

Next, round up the equipment you'll need. If you have access to a gym, it will probably have everything there. If you are doing this at home, there are good home substitutions you can use. Check in to www.healthykneescoach.com/shop to see a bundle of equipment that you can order.

If you want more help with starting than just this book, check out www.healthykneesforumula.com, our online program with videos, coaching, resources, and more.

2. I'm afraid I will make it worse
I bet that is one of the reasons you picked up this book. Because you are afraid of making it worse.

I want to reassure you that the best thing to do is follow the advice in this book and see how you feel. Follow the exercises in the order they are listed and do not move ahead until you feel like you are doing the first exercise well.

We laid out the program in an 8-week course, but for some people, it may take longer. That's okay! Do your best, see how you feel. Being muscle-sore is okay and a normal process of getting stronger.

We have tested this program for years—first on me, then, since 2015, with hundreds of students who've shown us that the program works to relieve pain, improve strength, and regain confidence in your movement.

Of course, we cannot guarantee that this program will work for everyone—there are too many conditions and circumstance combinations to account for.

We hope you will give it at least two weeks before deciding if it is or is not for you.

3. But I don't like working out

The exercise itself does not need to bring you joy, but it is necessary to get stronger.

Simply said, if you want the results, you have to do the work.

And if you just don't like workout out, it's time to reframe it. You are not just "working out" or just "lifting weights," you are <u>using the tools to make your body stronger and reduce your pain.</u> *You don't have to love it, but to get the results, you have to do it.*

It's like you are your own mechanic—you can't keep running a car with broken parts. You've got to fix it, and this is the simplest, most cost-effective way to get long term results.

And who knows? After you get in the habit of exercising two times per week, it may actually start to bring you more energy, better sleep, feeling stronger, and even a little bit of joy.

4. I'm too old to start something new

Now hold on, many studies have shown that weight training, even starting something new into your 90's (remember that study I mentioned?), has benefit for building strength and balance. Just take it slowly, master the move before you advance on to the next. The most important thing is to have good form as you do each strength move.

I think we all want good health at any age. We want to remain physically independent, and to do that, you need to be strong. Don't wait any longer; just get started (of course, seek your doctor's approval first).

5. I'm too out of shape to do this

The truth of the matter is that you must start where you are. You can't start anywhere else. You are not going to get in better shape without doing something to make a change. My recommendation is not to go crazy with getting started, but rather, be sensible. Commit to two workouts a week on consistent days and times. Make this a priority for yourself. YOU are important!

When that feels good, and you are ready, add in a third day per week to exercise. My formula is 2x/week strength training and 2x/week cardio (bicycling)—and it's the closest thing you'll ever get to a "magic pill." But work your way up to this! The Healthy Knees Formula program starts exactly that way—with 2X/week sessions—and helps you build from there.

6. Coaching is just for competitive athletes

We all could use another person who is on our side and rooting for us. A coach can help you recognize issues that may be standing in your way or help you find a way to fix them. Your coach can be your external eyes and ears, providing a different view of how you move and giving you feedback so you can make changes. I've had sports coaches and business coaches because I want to learn and improve. Your coach (that's this book!) provides you with a plan, so you don't have to spend years studying and researching the best way to do it. We've done that for you and condensed our best advice into this book.

7. What if I do it wrong?

Sometimes it is hard to know if you are doing things the right way, I get it. If any of the moves in this book cause you more pain, don't do them! You can start with the first part of the movement until just before that pain point. As you work on this range, you will get stronger.

But still, that nagging feeling exists—Am I doing it right? To provide you with more guidance, we go a step further in the Healthy Knees Formula program with access to videos showing you proper form. Plus, you'll have opportunities to chat with coaches in our weekly chat group. We are here to help and want you to have the best experience possible with the level of guidance you need.

Check it out at www.healthykneesformula.com

8. What if my mobility limits me?

We will start where you are. Do what you can without causing more pain. If you've been to physical therapy, keep up on the exercises they recommend and add in the ones from this book that feel good. This book is not meant to replace your doctor's advice or help from a physical therapist. It is meant to supplement that advice. If you are currently under the care of a health care professional, please check with them before adding exercises from this book.

9. I don't have the time

In the fitness business, this is an excuse I hear all of the time. Yes, you are busy. I get it. But the busiest, most successful people I know always take time to take care of themselves with regular exercise. Why? It makes you healthier and stronger, clears your mind, reduces stress, and gives you more energy so you can take better care of all the people and all the things in your life.

The people who tell me they don't have the time simply have not made exercise a priority in their life. Can you make time at lunch? Forego after-dinner TV? Can you get out of bed one hour earlier?

When my kids were young, and I was a stay-at-home working mom, my time to exercise was 5-6:30 am while my husband was home. Even though it was so darned early, it was MY time to make me a priority. I'd go to my gym for a spin class or weight training and come home with an accomplishment under my belt, feeling ready to tackle the day.

Here's the truth: In order to make time for exercise, you need to make it a priority and act on that priority. Make an "exercise appointment" for yourself on your calendar, phone, day timer—wherever you make your important appointments. Stick to it and don't let anything get in your way. Even on the days you don't feel like it, just show up! Do a little bit, and that little bit may just turn into a great workout.

10. Won't a knee surgery solve my problems?

Knee surgery can certainly solve some problems. And some problems can only be solved by surgery. But if you are weak, it won't solve that. If you are overweight and your joints are aching all of the time, surgery may not be the entire answer.

I believe that surgery should be looked at as the LAST strategy after you've done all of the strength training, cardio, and stretching that you can. There is a lot of new research showing that conservative therapy (exercise) has equal outcomes to surgery in a lot of (but not all) situations.

Besides, surgery is expensive! Not only from your own pocketbook, but recovery can be long and painful with missed work and is emotionally taxing. Wouldn't it be better to do the fitness work now and potentially avoid all of that pain, trauma, and fuss? The worst-case scenario is that you still may need surgery, but you go in stronger and will recover faster. That is a win for sure.

Surgery or not is ultimately a question for you to decide with the advice from your doctor.

To Sum it Up

What is your knee freedom worth to you? I know what it feels like to be limited in life because of knee pain. To look at a flight of stairs like they are your enemy. To give up the activities you love—running, skiing—because the pain is too much.

Working on strengthening your knees is about the quality of your life. It's about investing in yourself to avoid years of pain and disappointment.

I bet you'd like to live with knees that help propel you on to the exciting things in life. So, let's get going!

CHAPTER 7

MOVING FORWARD

Now it is time to take action! Here is the tough love part of this book: if you don't consistently do the work, you will not get the results. Simply owning this book will not help your knees. Now it is up to you to do the work.

1. What to do first

JUST. GET. STARTED.

Start where you are, follow the plan, and do what you can. There is nowhere else to begin.

The truth of the matter is that you are not going to make any changes in your knees unless you change something in your routine. Don't wait another minute; let's get started!

2. Mindset & Commitment

> *"Whether you think you can, or you think you can't—you're right."* —HENRY FORD

Having a mindset of success will help you along your path to making significant and meaningful changes in your own health and fitness. Yes, this will be a challenge, and for those of you who have never had a regular or consistent exercise plan as part of your life, this will be a big shift. **BUT IT IS NECESSARY and DO-ABLE** in order for you to get the results you are hoping for!

Let's start with a base commitment and make this part of your own operating system.

I want to make this as simple for you as possible. Here's your plan to get started:

SESSIONS PER WEEK: Your commitment is 2 days per week.

DAYS OF THE WEEK: Now, pick your days. Make them at least 48 hours apart, such as Monday and Wednesday, or Tuesday and Thursday, or Wednesday and Saturday... you get the idea.

TIME OF DAY: What time are you consistently going to exercise? Are you a morning person and want to do it first thing to get it out of the way and start with an accomplishment under your belt for the day? Or do you prefer a mid-morning or mid-afternoon time? Perhaps you'd rather take care of your exercise as a release right after work. Pick your time and stick to it.

Keep your two times per week schedule as your base. It becomes part of who you are. You can even say, "I'm the kind of person who always exercises a minimum of two times per week." What happens if you miss a day? The world will not end; you have not

ROBIN ROBERTSON | 123

failed. Just pick it right back up. The more days you miss, the harder it is to return to your newfound routine.

There may come a time in a month or two where you want to add in another day of strength training, and that is great! Go ahead and do that but be sure to schedule it just as you had your other two days.

RECORD YOUR COMMITMENT: Put it on your calendar, your phone, your fridge. Make these exercise appointments your top priority (because YOUR health IS that important)

SHARE YOUR COMMITMENT: Tell someone important to you about your plan: your spouse, your friends, your boss, your pet. Even better, get a buddy to do it with you so you can hold each other accountable.

3. Get pictures of all of the Exercises

Pictures, Pictures, Pictures—There were too many pictures to add to this book! And so, we've created a downloadable guide with pictures for every move that is FREE for you.

Simply go to: www.healthykneescoach.com/HKStrength and download your copy right now!

4. Get more help to make sure you are doing it right

The hardest part about starting a new exercise routine is knowing if you are doing it right and staying motivated. Results do not come overnight, and undoing years of toll on your bodies takes time. Healthy Knee Strength is the perfect place to start and is one of the key elements to caring for your knees.

WARNING: Here's what I DON'T want you to do: many people, when they start a new exercise routine, go from zero to 100% and plan to work out every day. While this might feel good for a short while, before they know it, they are burned out, overtired, and simply cannot sustain that level of effort. Their bodies are not getting the recovery they need. They are exhausted. They get hurt. And then they throw in the towel, stop exercising altogether, and say that it didn't work. It was simply way too much, too fast.

Please take my advice and start slowly. Two days per week are the minimum you need to start feeling and seeing change. If you are starting at zero exercise, stick with the two days per week for this entire 8-week program.

But if and when you want more, I invite you to join us in the Healthy Knees Formula program that takes this book to the next level with videos, print outs, weekly motivation, and weekly live questions and answers. You can ask the professionals if you are doing it right. The Healthy Knees Formula provides the long-term solution you've been hoping for so that you can do all the right things to help your knees feel great again.

FOR MORE HELP:
www.healthykneesformula.com
Additional Resources: (pictures for each exercise)
www.healthykneescoach.com/HKStrength

THANK YOU

Thank you so much for investing your time in reading this book. I hope it will serve as your guide to changing your knee health and returning to living life to the fullest.

If you have friends who also suffer from knee pain, please share this book with them!

We are always seeking to make our Healthy Knees programs better. I'd love to know how the information in this book helped you and if you have any suggestions for improvements. I invite you to write a review on Amazon, so others can know about your experience with this book.

Here's to your Healthy, Happy Knees!

Robin Robertson   Tyler Tobing

robin@healthykneescoach.com
Facebook: healthykneescoach
www.healthykneescoach.com

ROBIN ROBERTSON

Business Owner, Founder, Author

Since 2000, Robin Robertson and her husband Doug have owned and managed the Bellingham Training and Tennis Club in Bellingham, Washington. Robin is accomplished in a variety of training methods, including Functional Aging Specialist, ACE-certified personal trainer, USA Cycling Coach, author, and founder of Healthy Knees Coach.

Robin is a lifelong athlete who has had a total of 12 knee surgeries. She ran competitively in high school and college but turned to cycling to save her knees. Not daunted by poor knees, Robin toured the world on her bike and raced road bicycles. At ages 47 and 48, she was 2nd and 1st place Washington State Best All-Around Road Rider" Masters B Division and placed high in many other road racing events. She also raced mountain bikes, competing in the Leadville 100, among

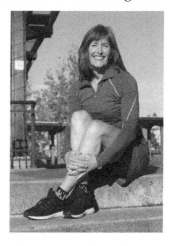

other events. She continues to train for cycling and fitness events, commutes to work, goes on multi-day, self-supported bicycle adventure tours, and rides her bike just for fun and to keep her knees in good health. When she's not on her bike or helping others to live healthy and active lives, Robin loves family time with her husband and two children and traveling to explore this amazing world.

TYLER BUDWEY

Fitness Director, Bellingham Training & Tennis Club

Tyler Budwey is a lifelong athlete, fitness advocate, and truth seeker. His exposure to sports, exercise, and injury in his high school and college career, as well as the help of a few quality educators, led him to seek out a career in the fitness world. Tyler received his Bachelor of Science in Exercise Physiology in 2016 and is an NCSA Certified Strength and Conditioning Specialist. Tyler started an internship at a physical therapy clinic in Massachusetts during his senior year of high school that became a job for the

next eight years. Tyler spent his time there working as a rehab aide, personal trainer, and high school strength and conditioning coach. This is where he blended his knowledge of the physical therapy world with that of sports performance.

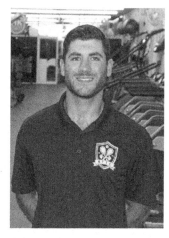

Tyler enjoys taking the knowledge he acquired working alongside physical therapists and applying it practically to the world of strength and conditioning. He takes the education of his clientele very seriously and is always aiming to deconstruct the myths surrounding exercise and fitness, that are all too rampant nowadays. Tyler continues to train not only for the health benefits, but also to support his wrestling, Jiu-jitsu, hiking, backpacking, mountain biking, and all-around mental wellbeing.

You can find out more about Robin, Tyler, Healthy Knees Coach, and the Bellingham Training and Tennis Club at the following:

www.healthykneescoach.com
www.betrainingtennis.com
Book: *Healthy Knees Cycling* (2015)
Book: *Healthy Knees Total Knee Replacement* (to be released 2020)

HEALTHYKNEESFORMULA.COM

We know you might be worried about doing things the right way, and that's why we created the Healthy Knees Formula for you.

This online program will help guide you every step of the way with a week by week coached program, so you know you are doing the right thing at the right time.

We know this isn't for everyone, because to get the results, you have to do the work. We've had hundreds of clients over the past five years of running this program who have successfully reduced or eliminated their knee pain and are back to living the life they love. We think you should have this chance too.

OUR FULL HEALTHY KNEES FORMULA PROGRAM INCLUDES:
Stage 1: Knee Resolve—Starting where you are with a strength-building program to stabilize your knee and stop the downward spiral.

Stage 2: Knee Relief—Reduce pain through strength training + cycling foundation to build your base.

Stage 3: Knee Rebuilding—Build strength through muscular development + cycling for knee mobility and stamina.

Stage 4: Knee Restore—Become powerful with a sense of knee freedom through a higher level of cycling and strength training.

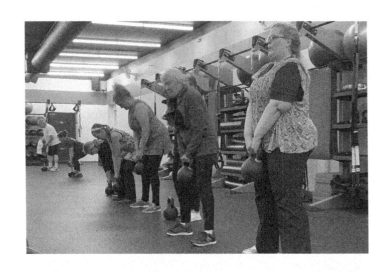

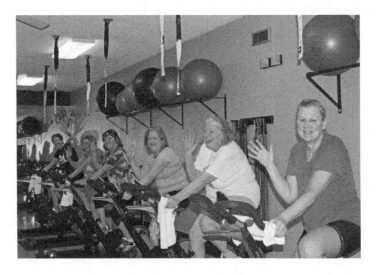

Excited to get started?

Visit us at healthykneesformula.com

Made in the USA
Columbia, SC
04 June 2020

98440851R00085